PROBLEM-BASED LEARNING
APPLIED TO
M____ _ EDUCATION

By

HOWARD S. BARROWS, MD

Revised Edition published 2000
Former title: Practice-Based Learning: Problem-Based Learning
Applied to Medical Education

Published by
Southern Illinois University School of Medicine
Springfield, Illinois

ISBN – 0.931369-34-7
Library of Congress (94-065480)
First Edition

Revised Edition published 2000
Former title: Practice-Based Learning: Problem-Based Learning
Applied to Medical Education

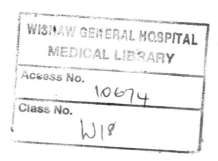

This book is dedicated to
the memory of

JAMES E. ANDERSON MD

An unsung hero in medical education.
A phenomenal educator and tutor who originated the idea of small
group, problem-based learning at McMaster University.

ACKNOWLEDGEMENTS

Linda Distlehorst and LuAnn White have reviewed portions of this book. My wife Phyllis has reviewed it in its entirety and made many valuable suggestions in both grammar and clarity. Rosemary Beiermann has engineered all of the complexities of reorganization required to bring this revised edition to fruition. I am indebted to all of these people. What failings this edition may still have are totally of my doing.

TABLE OF CONTENTS

Introduction vii

Background ix

1. Authentic Problem-Based Learning 1

2. The Goals Of Undergraduate Medical Education . . . 4

3. The Challenge Of The Patient's Problem 7

4. The Physician's Clinical Reasoning Process 12

5. The Clinical Reasoning Process is only Part of
    the Process In Solving The Patient's Problem 23

6. Self-Directed Learning 30

7. The Educational Objectives That Are Addressed By
    Problem-Based Learning 33

8. The Curricular Requirements of Problem-Based
    Learning 37

9. The Authentic Problem-Based Learning Process . . 48

10. The Authentic Problem-Based Learning Process
    (continued) 67

11. The Authenticity of Problem-Based Learning 81

12. Two Common Concerns of Medical Teachers 85

13. Integrating Other Learning Methods into Problem-
    Based Learning 89

14. Variables That Can Alter the Effectiveness of
    Problem-Based Learning 91

15. Assessment in Problem-Based Learning 98

16. Applying Problem-Based Learning
    to the Clerkship Years 111

17.   Converting to Problem-Based Learning 117

18.   Choosing Problems 121

19.   Evaluating The Effectiveness Of Problem-Based
        Learning as an Instructional Method 125

20.   Criteria for Analyzing a Problem-Based
        Learning Curriculum 130

Appendix I 134

Appendix II 137

References 140

Index   146

INTRODUCTION

This book is designed for medical teachers who wish to consider problem-based learning as an educational method to be used in their courses or curriculum in medical school. It is also designed for those teachers who have made that decision but would like to have guidelines for the design and development of a problem-based curriculum.

My two prior books, *Problem-based Learning; an approach to medical education* (1980, co-authored by Robyn Tamblyn) and *How to Design a Problem-based Curriculum for the Preclinical Years* (1985) have been used extensively by teachers interested in problem-based learning but are now out of date. Much more has been learned through the experience of many more schools that have undertaken this method and from an increasing number of studies related to problem-based learning.

Problem-based learning has now been applied to many areas including education for other professions and higher education, and is now being extensively developed in secondary education. As a consequence of its being widely adopted, the meaning of the term problem-based learning has become clouded and confused. I've chosen the term *Authentic problem-based Learning* as it provides the orientation and focus for the design of problem-based learning in medicine so that it will be most effective in preparing medical students for their professional roles as physicians, the center of which is the practice of medicine. The rationale for this term will be expanded on in the first chapter.

This book is based on my own continuing work and experience with problem-based learning both as a member of a medical school faculty actively involved in problem-based learning and on consultations and workshops working with teachers in many different schools.

Although this book starts with problem-based learning in the basic science or preclinical years as preparation for the clinical clerkships, the extension of problem-based learning to the clinical clerkships is also considered. *The Tutorial Process*[1] describing the skills required of the tutor was written as a companion to this book.

BACKGROUND

The original problem-based curriculum at McMaster University, featuring small learning groups with a faculty tutor, was established thirty years ago.[2,3] As a newly created school, McMaster began with this revolutionary problem-based curriculum after a reasonably luxurious four-year opportunity to set it up. A few years later two more new schools, widely spaced across the globe one at Maastricht University in the Netherlands and the other at University of Newcastle in Australia, undertook problem-based learning curricula. There was much cross-fertilization between all three schools. Many faculty from Maastricht and Newcastle spent months to years at McMaster as they were planning their curricula.

Over twenty years ago the University of New Mexico School of Medicine created another problem-based learning revolution by establishing an alternative, problem-based curriculum emphasizing rural, primary care. It was designed for a small number of students and ran parallel with their traditional curriculum. The initial development of this curriculum was financed by an external grant from the Kellogg Foundation and required changes in curriculum design and teaching that were quite different from their traditional curriculum. Promoting this new method for teaching students among the faculty was a new and difficult challenge for the small, dedicated, alternative curriculum faculty at New Mexico.[4] They were pioneers in creating the change from traditional to problem-based curricula. Subsequently, other medical schools such as Harvard, Bowman Gray, Rush and Southern Illinois University established alternative, parallel curricula and faced the challenge of faculty and curriculum conversion.

Over the last decade, many new and developing countries around the world have also initiated problem-based curricula.[5] More recently, several schools including Harvard and Sherbrooke University in Canada have converted their entire, previously conventional, curricula to problem-based learning.[6,7] The University of Kentucky School of Medicine developed a problem-based learning curriculum in surgery and more recently problem-based learning has been incorporated in psychiatry and surgical clerkships at Southern Illinois University. A 1991 Curriculum Directory of the Association of American Medical Colleges suggested that over ninety medical schools in the USA are now considering problem-based learning in some form or other or in some part of their curricula.[8] At this point problem-based learning cannot be considered as an experimental method in medical education. It has probably been more thoroughly studied and evaluated than have the traditionally accepted educational methods used in medical school. Those teachers who have undertaken the change to problem-based learning usually have done so on the basis of a personal educational philosophy that was in line with problem-based learning or out of concern for their school's curriculum and teaching methods. To many faculty, medical students seem bored and dissatisfied with their experience in medical school and consider the basic science years as a difficult and irrelevant hurdle that has to be passed to become a doctor. There is too much emphasis on memorization of facts for their own sake, and students seem to readily forget what they were taught later in their clinical years. External pressure to rid the curriculum of the need to provide comprehensive coverage of the content in all disciplines basic to medicine and to make the first two years of medical school more relevant to the practice of medicine has come from medical school deans, university presidents and, more recently, from the Liaison Committee for Medical Education during its review of medical schools. This pressure has also provided impetus towards problem-based learning. Often a personal encounter with problem-based learning either as an observer in an educational workshop or visiting a problem-based school has also stimulated medical teachers' interest in changing to problem-based learning.

The many studies that have been carried out to evaluate the effectiveness of problem-based learning are fraught with problems that make them difficult to interpret. There are uncontrolled variables in the educational setting that could affect student performance independent of problem-based learning. Many studies have insufficient numbers of subjects. They use limited or inappropriate assessment tools such as scores on the National Board of Examiner's United States Medical Licensing Examination (USMLE) step I that do not measure the educational objectives addressed by problem-based learning. In some programs there is a possible bias produced by admission policies (do the "better", older, more mature students tend to volunteer for problem-based learning?). A number of reviews of the literature dealing with the evaluation of problem-based learning have been published.[9,10,11] The results of these papers will be discussed in more detail in Chapter XIX. Now that problem-based learning curricula have increased significantly, and larger numbers of physicians are now going into practice that are products of problem-based learning, there are studies underway that will continue to provide additional data.[12, 73]

Many early studies compared the scores achieved on National Board of Medical Examiners Part I (now replaced by the USMLE Step I) taken after completing the first two basic science years. Overall, no truly significant differences have been found with these scores. However, this examination does not measure competencies or skills that are important or central to the rationale for employing problem-based learning. The results only assure the skeptic that problem-based learning is doing no harm in terms of the range and extent of knowledge that students in both curricula can recall.

The many teachers and the increasing number of schools that have adopted problem-based learning have done so on the basis of the logic behind its use and the fact that it has provided an exciting and motivating way for students to learn. Many students contemplating entering medical school are now selecting schools on the basis of whether they offer a problem-based learning curriculum. As mentioned previously, medical students have become jaded and bored with preclinical years made up of endless lectures by a parade of faculty and the need to memorize endless facts for their own sake just to pass examinations that ask for regurgitation of memorized facts. Students are required to memorize incredible amounts of information to survive.[13]

Unfortunately most of the reviewers who have attempted to synthesize the results of studies evaluating problem-based learning do not realize how difficult it is to generalize from reports and studies from individual schools that claim to use problem-based learning. In fact, most medical teachers are unaware of the many marked dif-

ferences that are present in these schools and how erroneous it can
be to generalize about problem-based learning from observations or
reports from a particular school. PBL curricula can differ remarkably
in curricular design, the extent of the curriculum that is problem-
based (all years, first two years, alternative, parallel track or entire
curriculum), the problem formats used by students (printed cases,
vignettes, simple to complex simulations), the role of the tutor, the
size of the student group, the degree to which conventional curricula
compete with problem-based learning, the kinds and number of
subjects or disciplines that are not included in the problem-based
learning curriculum (anatomy and biochemistry, for example, are
often taught in a conventional manner in some schools with problem-based learning), the degree to which students are given responsibility for their learning as opposed to the teacher, the stress put
on self-directed learning or clinical problem solving, the methods
used for student assessment (multiple choice questions versus per-
formance-based assessments), and the use of grades versus pass-fail
decisions. The results of a detailed questionnaire by Kelson and
Distlehorst sent to all schools who claim to be using problem-based
learning underline the fact that problem-based learning can be a
meaningless term unless what goes on in a curriculum is clearly
defined.[14]

This book will build the case for a well developed and researched
type of problem-based learning that has evolved through twenty-
five years of design - application - assessment - and redesign. It represents problem-based learning in its more rigorous and pure form.
Understanding this particular species and the rationale for all the
elements in its design, should give you sufficient background to
design a problem-based learning curriculum based on sound educational principles. One that reflects both the particular objectives
and expectations you, or your school, has for the medical students
it graduates and the resources within your school.

The basic sciences of education are educational psychology and
cognitive science. The information from these fields is as essential
to educational practice as are the basic sciences of anatomy, physiology, etc. to the practice of medicine. In the light of these sciences,
it could be considered educational malpractice to expose students
to all the information you may feel is essential from your discipline

and then test them at the end of the course to see if they are able to regurgitate a sufficient amount of that information in an oral or written test. Many studies have shown that the students will forget most of what you have asked them to memorize and will not be able to apply what they can recall in practice. This is not only educational malpractice, it is tragically inefficient when you consider how much energy faculty put into teaching and students put into studying during these preclinical years to result in such a small yield.

The particular way in which students are asked to learn has a strong influence on how well they will be able to recall and apply what they have learned in the real clinical world outside of the medical school. If your major concern as a teacher is only that students do well on written tests of recognition and recall, the educational approach just described will accomplish that. However, if you expect your students to:
- Become independent
- Reason their way through patient problems
- Recall and apply what they have been taught in medical school to the care of their patients
- Recognize when their skills and knowledge are not adequate to the clinical task they are confronting and
- Acquire new information and skills as they need it, and, as medical research moves ahead, keeping contemporary in their knowledge and skills

Then the conventional medical education approach, described previously, is inappropriate.

Over the last thirty years there has been a growing body of research in these sciences basic to education that provides information essential to well thought out educational practice. Much of this information is incorporated in the problem-based learning method described here. Schmidt, Norman and Myers have provided overviews of the many studies in psychology and cognition that have underlined the scientific basis for problem-based learning in general.[15,16,17]

The first chapters will elaborate further on the background for a well designed problem-based learning curriculum by considering the goals of undergraduate medical education, the challenge patient problems present, the nature of the physician's clinical reasoning process, how that process is associated with knowledge needed to care for patients, and the importance of self-directed learning for an effective career in medicine. The remaining chapters will deal with the design of an effective problem-based learning curriculum

Chapter One

AUTHENTIC PROBLEM-BASED LEARNING

The problem-based learning method described here had its origins in simulations of patient problems called "problem boxes" that were developed for medical students on a neurological clerkship at the University of Southern California in 1969. These problems were designed to extend the experience of clinical clerks to patient problems that might not be available to them on the hospital service during any particular rotation. The problem box contained, among other things, a booklet that would disclose the patient problem to the student in small segments. At the end of each segment the student was asked to decide on the questions he or she might ask the patient and, later, on the items of the physical and neurological examination that should be performed. The boxes also contained film loops that would allow the student to see the patient being examined and photographs of x-rays, funduscopic appearances, pathology slides, etc. as appropriate. In 1973 the Project for Learning Resources Design (PLRD) was established at McMaster to further develop problem simulation formats for problem-based learning that would encourage the development of clinical reasoning skills.[18,19] As the problem box did not allow the student to inquire freely about the patient problem, as occurs in clinical practice, alternative formats such as the "P4," a card deck that permitted free inquiry, were developed. The activities of the PLRD group inevitably led to concerns about the skills of the tutor in using problem formats and the appropriate design of problem-based learning curricula. Over seven years, a ten-week neuroscience block in the McMaster curriculum was used as a laboratory school by the PLRD for the application and evaluation of problem formats, tutor techniques and curriculum design.[20,21,22,23,24,25] In its last four years, the ten-week block was given four times a year (the one hundred students in each year were divided into "schools" of 25) allowing the PLRD to carry out developmental work with twenty iterations of the course. The emphasis on the development of clinical reasoning skills along with problem-solving and self-directed learning skills began to define the unique character of this particular species of problem-based learning. The PLRD initiated weeklong workshops for tutors that were attended by faculty members from other schools interested in developing problem-based learning.[26] Visitors to McMaster, interested in problem-based learning were invariably scheduled to work with the PLRD and to observe its neuroscience course. As a result, this particular method was adopted and adapted by teachers from other schools.

This particular problem-based learning approach and its associated problem formats has been further developed and applied at Southern Illinois University Medical School, initially in problem-based learning workshops and materials for teachers from other schools and, in the last ten years, in the school's parallel or alternative problem-based learning curriculum.[27,28,29]

As there are so many different varieties of problem-based learning, it would be helpful to give this particular method a name that distinguishes it from the others. However, since any unique name applied to problem-based learning should point to its distinctive features, the term *Authentic Problem-Based Learning* is used in this book. In education, an authentic education requires the learner to go through the same activities during learning that are valued in the real world. This species of problem-based learning was given the adjective authentic for the following reasons:

1) This problem-based learning method is designed to help students develop the reasoning process used by physicians in their clinical practice as they reason through the patient problem: generating hypotheses; carrying out an inquiry through history and physical; analyzing data obtained from the patient; synthesizing the data into a meaningful picture of the patient's problem; and making diagnostic and therapeutic decisions. [30]

2) Problem simulation formats are used that present actual patient problems to students in the same manner that occurs in practice. The formats are designed to permit the student to inquire freely on history, carry out any part of the physical examination and order any laboratory tests in any sequence as occurs in practice.

3) The sequence of behaviors required of the student as they work with patient problems and carry out self-directed learning is the same sequence of behaviors that is required in clinical practice and described in chapters IX and X.

4) The patient problems selected in the curriculum are based on actual patients and represent the frequent and important problems that will appear in practice, again underlining authenticity. The problems in a problem-based learning curriculum, taken together, form the curriculum. This ensures that the information from the basic and clinical sciences that the students will learn in their problem related work is an up-to-date and relevant curriculum for students preparing for the practice of medicine.

The intent of authentic problem-based learning is to challenge the learner with patient problems and other problems that will be faced in practice both as a stimulus for learning and a focus for organizing what has been learned for later recall and application to future clinical work.

There are many tasks, such as the well baby examination, work on medical teams, community health problem, educating patients and the community, and problems relating to managed care that are also appropriate challenges of learning. The term "problem" is often considered too narrowly as only referring to ill patients. These are not the only problems that physicians face in their practice. These other problems should also be in the problem-based learning curriculum.

Chapter Two

THE GOALS OF UNDERGRADUATE MEDICAL EDUCATION

Before undertaking any enterprise or innovation, it is essential to know what your objectives are or what it is you hope to accomplish so that the enterprise can be appropriately designed to achieve what it is you expect. Stated objectives provide expected outcomes that will allow you, and anyone else, to determine whether the enterprise is successful. The obvious objective of any medical school curriculum is to produce a competent physician. Therefore, faculty teachers contemplating curriculum design or review should carefully consider what are the characteristics of the physician they want their curriculum to produce. The methods selected in any undergraduate curriculum should emphasize the development of those abilities, skills and attitudes desired in the graduate—a physician about to enter post-graduate training where there is heavy responsibility and far less supervision in the care of patients. The rationale for problem-based learning as an educational method and the possible inappropriateness of more traditionally used methods in undergraduate medical education become apparent when the goals for the graduating medical students are considered.

It is beyond the scope of this book to attempt separation of the goals for undergraduate medical education from postgraduate education. And, it is usually a pointless undertaking as many medical students graduate into postgraduate residency programs that are not under the control of the medical school. It would be ideal and much more efficient of time and effort to be able to design an appropriate curriculum that continued without a break until students were to enter practice. In other words enter as a medical student and exit as a physician ready to practice. The objectives considered here are for the mythical, undifferentiated physician about to enter any primary, secondary or tertiary care specialty. Appropriately then, this is only a most basic set of core expectations for what medicine as a profession (and the public) might expect of a physician and considered as objectives for undergraduate medical education. These basic, core expectations or goals will do well as a basis for you to consider the appropriateness of problem-based learning.

Your medical school should augment and elaborate on these objectives to match their particular expectations and values.

Basic, non-negotiable expectations for the performance of physicians

There are at least two basic, non-negotiable expectations that the public has a right to expect of physicians.

1) Physicians should be able to manage the health problems of the patients for which they become responsible in an effective, efficient and humane manner.

> "Effective" management means that physicians' diagnoses must be accurate and sufficiently refined to facilitate the choice of an appropriate management plan. The management plans chosen must be designed to provide the most effective relief possible, to improve the patient's prognosis over no treatment, to be the best for the particular patient among alternative therapies, and to meet the expectations and needs of the patient with the least risk, cost, and unnecessary discomfort.

> "Efficient" means that physicians' management of the patient must be cost effective and avoids unnecessary treatments and tests, and the use of unnecessary health personnel or facilities. This aspect of physician performance becomes even more important in the national and international trends towards controlling health care costs and providing health care for all.

> "Humane" means that physicians must have effective interpersonal and communication skills. They must be able to work with patients in a way that will invoke confidence, trust, and satisfaction. The care of the patient must be sensitive to the patient's particular concerns, values, needs, cultural and family setting, and financial situation.

2) Continue learning throughout their professional lives to meet the often unique and changing needs of patients and the problems

they present, the changing problems and demands in the health care system, and to keep contemporary in medical knowledge and practice.

> The increasing complexities of diagnostic and therapeutic tools, the ever expanding knowledge about diseases and disease processes, the increasingly complex issues of ethical and moral decisions related to these advances and the dramatic changes in health care delivery systems coupled with rapid changes in information access and handling make the task of self-education essential to the practice of medicine.

There is no question that physicians should have a rich and extensive knowledge base in order to practice medicine and you might be distressed that this obviously important goal is not stated as a primary objective. However, it is of no value to have physicians who have their heads packed full of facts but who either can't recall them or apply them to the care of their patients. The existence of an encyclopedic knowledge base in a physician's head provides no assurance that that knowledge will be recalled and used effectively in the care of patients. A statement that physicians should have a rich and extensive knowledge base stated as a free standing objective does not underline the concern that the knowledge should be applied in order to be of any value. Such an objective could be satisfied by a good performance on a written or oral examination. However, if you reason through the implications of the first objective, it should be clear that the quality of patient care specified requires an extensive but useable knowledge base. Good performances by physicians in caring for their patients automatically indicates the possession of an adequate knowledge base, whereas, the possession of a good knowledge base does not indicate a good clinical performance. The first objective requires an appropriate foundation of knowledge in medicine and the sciences basic to medicine.

These non-negotiable, most basic, core objectives are not intended to be complete, as there are many other objectives that any medical faculty would and should add to the list. As the basic objectives for physician performance they will do us well in considering problem-based learning.

Chapter Three

THE CHALLENGE OF THE PATIENT'S PROBLEM

I f we want to produce physicians who are able to reason through a patient problem effectively and efficiently, the characteristics of patient problems that challenge physician reasoning need to be understood so that the rationale for designing problem simulations that support inquiry, and the rationale for the procedures followed in the tutorial group by the tutor and learners can be appreciated.

Characteristics of patient problems

When the patient is first encountered there is usually insufficient information available for a physician to decide on a diagnosis and a plan of care.

More information than is initially available is needed for the physician to understand what is most likely responsible for the patient's problem and to decide on what actions may be required to provide relief and/or resolution.

Most patients present with just a complaint, and it is obvious that more information will have to be obtained by the physician initially through history and physical examination and subsequently through laboratory tests to come to a working diagnosis(es) and a treatment plan. In fact, no matter how much information may be present when the physician first encounters the patient (medical records, referral letters, prior laboratory results), the physician will always want more information on history, physical examination and from additional laboratory tests in order to come to a diagnostic impression and to decide on management. Presenting students with patient problems that contain most of the information needed (such as in case vignettes or case histories) is inconsistent with the challenge they will face in practice. Physicians have to obtain the needed additional information for diagnosis and treatment through a hypothetico-deductive inquiry process (described in Chapter IV). This is a point missed by those who think physicians diagnose through pattern recognition, comparing the pattern of the patient's problem with patterns of diagnostic entities recalled in the mind. Initially, the patient does not present with any pattern that will allow comparison with patterns entertained by the physician. Physicians need to fill out the patient's presenting picture with more information on history and physical examination to create a pattern that can be compared with those in their mind to verify or eliminate diagnostic possibilities. Another point that should be recognized is that the real challenge to the physician in practice is the patient problem that does not fit into any diagnostic pattern.

There is no one right way for the physician to get the additional information needed.

If different physicians are given the same patient problem (as can be done with studies using standardized patients) each will go about getting the additional information in different ways. Although there may be a core of common questions and examinations performed by all of them, each will ask different questions in a different order, perform different items on the physical examination in different ways and sequences, and even order different laboratory tests. Despite these differences, they will often come up with similar diagnoses and treatment plans. Physicians have differing patient and educational experiences in their long-term memory banks. These produce unique configurations of data about the diagnoses they entertain and different experiences with what works to make a diagnosis and decide on treatment. As a consequence, each physician requires somewhat different information to support or deny the diagnostic ideas entertained. This means that physicians have to inquire, explore and probe in their own way, based on past experiences and education, to get the information needed to fill out the picture of the patient to establish a diagnosis (as well as a differential diagnosis) and treatment plan.

As new information is obtained, the patient's problem may change and become quite different than was suspected at the beginning of the encounter.

As suggested by the first characteristic, the way the patient presents is not unlike the treachery presented to mariners by the tip of the iceberg above the surface of the water that gives no indication as to the extent, shape or size of the iceberg under water. As the physician begins to inquire and new data are added to the patient's picture, it may become more complex or serious than suspected, involve different or multiple organ systems, and possibly involve significant medical or psychosocial complications that were unsuspected.

Despite the most careful and complete investigation of the patient's problem and even with the most straightforward of patient problems, the physician can never be certain that the diagnoses decided upon are correct and that the management plan chosen represents the best decision.

Important data that a physician might like to have to verify a diagnosis or make a treatment decision may not be available from the patient for a variety of reasons. Data obtained from the patient on history and physical examination may be conflicting and ambiguous or communication with the patient may be difficult. With many diseases, there are not enough characteristic symptoms and signs or definitive laboratory tests to confirm a diagnosis with certainty, and the commonest of diseases can present in unusual ways. Even in what seems to be a straightforward case there can be an unsuspected diagnosis responsible, or an unsuspected complication present. Despite all of this, the physician has to make decisions and take action. The patient's problem cannot be set aside for another day when the problem might be easier to understand or until medical science can provide better diagnostic tests or better defined treatment guidelines. Unlike problem solving in other professions or in scientific investigations, the physician has to provide care for the patient at the time, despite the fact that there is a chance of being wrong.

These four preceding characteristics are not unique to patients as a problem. They are the characteristics of what cognitive psychologists refer to as "ill-structured" problems. Most of the problems we all face at work and in our lives are ill-structured and have the same characteristics:

1) more information is needed than is immediately available to understand the problem,

2) there is no one right way to get this information; the problem solver has to question, explore, observe, probe, and experiment to get further information,

3) the problem often changes as new information is acquired,

4) the problem solver can never be sure the analysis of the problem or the solution or action taken to resolve the problem is the right one

Personality factors such as attitudes, emotions and hidden agendas add additional ill-structuredness to patient problems as they present to the physician (and the problems clients or customers present to other professions). Therefore, patient problems, as ill-structured problems, take on this fifth characteristic.

The patient is a necessary and important partner in the diagnostic and treatment process.

The quality or value of data obtained by the physician from history and physical examination is dependent on the patient's ability to understand, communicate and cooperate. The effectiveness of treatment also depends on the patient's understanding, cooperation, emotional state and ability to communicate. Cooperation and communication can be affected by a multitude of factors that may be beyond the control of the physician and can tax the physician's communication skills such as the patient's level of consciousness, mental aberrations, or ability to speak in English. However, many of the factors that do affect cooperation and communication are within the physician's control and depend on clinical and interpersonal skills.

The patient expects to receive professional service from the physician and expects care and understanding. A frightened, hostile, unhappy or confused patient will not communicate or cooperate as well during assessment or comply with the treatment plan as well as a reassured patient who understands the care being offered, and is satisfied with that care. It is not sufficient for the physician to have good technical and problem-solving skills to care for patients. Interpersonal, communication, and patient-education skills are equally as essential.

With these characteristics of patient problems in mind, we now need to look at how the problem-solving process (the clinical reasoning process) of the effective, efficient and humane physician can effectively deal with the challenges patient problems offer.

Chapter Four

THE PHYSICIAN'S CLINICAL REASONING PROCESS

The use of patient problem simulations designed to help the students practice their clinical reasoning skills and a tutorial process aimed at helping students develop clinical reasoning skills is one of the defining characteristic of authentic problem-based learning. It is important that the physician's clinical reasoning process is understood in some detail. The process is well suited to deal effectively with the ill-structured problem patients present.

There have been many studies of the physician's clinical reasoning process. Most have shown that physicians encountering an unfamiliar, difficult or complex problem use a "hypothetico-deductive" reasoning process.[31,32,33,34,35] The significance of the modifiers "unfamiliar, difficult or complex" is important, as expert physicians who work repetitively with the usual and straightforward problems in their fields tend to take shortcuts. This happens after working through similar problems many times using the hypothetico-deductive process, and shortcuts become almost automatic. We all take shortcuts with repetitive problems, no longer thinking through all possibilities but plunging into what we know is the heart of the matter. Unfortunately, this "forward thinking", as it is sometimes called, can lead to error if the problem encountered has unusual features that were not detected in the physician's forward reasoning shortcut. The students in the undergraduate curriculum are amateurs; expertise and forward thinking will only come later with the accumulated experience of the clinical clerkship, postgraduate and practice years.

Although it is reassuring that studies of physician reasoning all tend to confirm the use of this hypothetico-deductive reasoning process, it is even more reassuring to see that the hypothetico-deductive process is the logical process to effectively deal with the challenges offered by the patient's ill-structured problem.

The following stages are identifiable in the hypothetico-deductive process. The manner in which this problem-solving skill used by the physician manages the challenge of the patient's problem will be stressed with each stage. This emphasizes the importance of acquiring this complex skill in medical school to ensure that the graduate can provide effective, efficient care to patients. What follows here is described in more detail elsewhere.[30]

The relationship of medical knowledge to the reasoning skills of the physician is discussed in the next chapter. This will emphasize the importance of learning this skill in the very beginning of medical school while basic science information is being learned. This is central to the logic and effectiveness of problem-based learning.

Much of this reasoning activity occurs quickly and almost unconsciously in the thinking of experienced physicians. However, on reflection, most will recognize the presence of these steps in their own thinking.

Generation of multiple hypotheses

As soon as the physician listens to the patient's initial complaint and has asked a few questions to clarify it, he or she almost automatically generates hypotheses. The hypotheses are brought to mind by associations with the patient's complaint combined with a number of observations such as the patient's sex, age, manner and body habitus. These hypotheses can be specific diagnostic entities, syndromes, anatomical, physiological or pathological entities that, in the physician's mind, could be explanations of the patient problem. These mental entities have been called hypotheses, prototypes, schemata, patterns, hunches, ideas, etc. Whatever they are called, each represents a label in the mind of the physician for a collection of facts about an illness that are recalled in the physician's mind. Usually two to five hypotheses are generated. Among them is the worst case scenario possible with that patient's complaint, even if remote, as it cannot be overlooked. The other hypotheses usually represent likely conditions that are treatable. Feltovich, Johnson, et al describes the collected hypotheses of the expert physician as a "logical competitor set."[36] This nicely characterizes the hypotheses generated as those that compete as possible, logical explanations for the patient's problem and suggest the kind of information that needs to be obtained from the patient through inquiry.

As a group, these hypotheses generated in the physician's mind at the outset of the patient encounter set the boundaries for the physician's search for more information. Since, as pointed out in the first characteristic of a patient problem, there is not enough information initially present for the physician to be able to diagnose and care for the patient; a guide is needed to determine what additional information is needed. The potential boundaries for information about a patient problem are enormous, and hours could be spent asking all questions possible of the patient and performing every item of the physical examination. This would be impractical and tedious. Hypotheses provide the physician with guidelines or focus for the kinds of information on history and physical examination that would be of most benefit in establishing diagnostic and treatment decisions.

Hypothesis generation is a creative aspect of patient problem solving. It is an inductive, lateral thinking activity used by the physician to think of the possible conditions that might be suggested by the patient's problem. It is here that new and unique ideas about patient problems can be developed.

Inquiry strategy

Using the hypotheses that were generated as a guide, the physician carries out an inquiry to obtain more data from the patient that will support or weaken the hypotheses considered. The brunt of this inquiry is through history taking. The physician inquires about those symptoms that would be expected with the hypotheses considered as well as symptoms that would tend to separate alternative hypotheses being considered in the logical competitor set. This is disciplined, logical, vertical, deductive, problem-oriented reasoning. One study of physicians' reasoning showed that they obtained nearly three fourths of the information they would need to make a diagnosis before the patient encounter was half over.[33] An efficient inquiry strategy is essential in emergencies or when time is limited, as it often is in the real world of practice, and there is not the luxury of an extended time to ask many possible questions.

Interspersed with this problem-oriented inquiry is a menu-oriented inquiry used when the physician wishes to get background information about the patient's prior health and family history, and to uncover other possible symptoms related to different organ systems that could suggest problems other than those suspected. This inquiry does not require careful, deductive reasoning and is mostly a matter of memorizing lists of questions. This menu-driven inquiry is also used by physicians to give them time to ponder the patient's problem and consider what other hypotheses or inquiry needs to be undertaken. The experienced physician usually restricts menu-driven inquiry to those questions that involve the organ systems that could be involved in the patient's problem. Menu-driven inquiry is severely attenuated in emergencies when every action should count and the luxury of time is not available.

The same problem-oriented and menu-driven inquiry can be seen in the physical examination. It is a common observation that 95% of the diagnosis is made on the history. The physical examination is often limited by physicians to those items that would confirm the diagnosis being considered or to separate competing hypotheses.

In many medical settings today the number of patients seen in a given time determines the income to the physician, the practice, or health organization in which the physician practices. Asking numerous irrelevant questions with a menu-driven inquiry and performing unnecessary items on the physical examination wastes time for the physician and the patient and wastes money.

The value of good inquiry skills looms even larger in the ordering of laboratory and diagnostic tests to further the investigation of the patient. Here incisive, problem-oriented inquiry is essential in ordering only those tests that are needed and in the right sequence to substantiate the hypothesis being considered. This inquiry should be coupled with knowledge of test sensitivity and specificity. Efficient reasoning here can significantly cut the costs of patient care.

As described before, with the ill-structured problems patients present, more information needs to be obtained to understand the problem and there is no one right way to get that information. With the hypotheses as a guide to the information needed and the use of deductive inquiry to get the information that should identify the most likely of the hypotheses, the ill-structured problem can be efficiently and effectively tackled.

Data analysis

As the patient provides answers to questions asked and findings are obtained from the physical examination, new information beyond that initially present becomes available to the physician. The physician analyzes this new information against the hypotheses entertained. Does it strengthen, substantially weaken or eliminate any of the hypotheses being considered or does it suggest new and unsuspected hypotheses?

Data synthesis (the "illness script")

When the ongoing analysis of newly obtained information reveals information that may be significant in relationship to the hypotheses under consideration or seems significant in understanding or treating the patient's problem; it is added to the information the physician is accumulating in his or her mind about the patient problem. This growing mental representation of the patient's problem is more than just a collection of the important facts learned about the patient during history and physical examination. They are organized by the physician in a cause and effect relationship that suggests the chain of events that led to the patient's problem and the pathophysiologic or psychobiological mechanism's responsible. This organized mental representation has been referred to in studies of physician cognition as an "illness script."[37,38] This growing mental synthesis records the present and changing shape of the structure of the patient's problem as described in the third characteristic of a patient problem. It is a vehicle for communication between physicians. In describing a patient problem to another physician for consultation or for fresh ideas, the physician presents this synthesis or script in a concise form. On hearing it, the other physician incorporates that synthesis and generates hypotheses based on her or his different experiences or expertise and then asks, in effect, "Have you thought of so and so?" (hypothesis) or, "Did you ask such and such a question or perform such and such examination or test?" (inquiry strategy) The lack of an illness script in the minds of clerks or residents giving an oral presentation of a patient's case is a frustrating experience for the clinical teacher as it makes his presentation sound like an unfathomable jumble of facts.

These are elements of the clinical reasoning seen as the physician reasons through the patient's ill-structured problem: inductive reasoning followed by deductive reasoning (hypotheses/inquiry); analysis and synthesis.

This is not a linear process as might be suggested by this description. Inquiry may lead to a blind alley ,and new hypotheses need to be generated. Menu-driven inquiry may need to be employed to find new clues about the problem when problem-based inquiry fails to substantiate the hypotheses considered. An unsuspected finding may suggest new hypotheses. The initial hypotheses may be too broad in scope to initiate any treatment and more refined ones need to be generated to carry the inquiry further.

Diagnostic and treatment decisions

At some point physicians have to come to a decision about their diagnosis and management. The time in the encounter it takes to do this relates to the time the physicians have available and the urgency of the patient's situation. Many activities can be sacrificed with time pressure; such as, chatting with the patient to get to know him or her as a person; checking into family and personal demographics; reviewing the patient's symptoms again to be sure they are understood; and carrying out a careful review of systems. The decisions to end the encounter are also determined by the impression that no more helpful data can be obtained from the patient during the present encounter, or that enough data has been obtained to make diagnostic and treatment decisions.

Despite all the ambiguities that might be present and the lack of data to be more certain, physicians have to make a decision and act. As mentioned previously, there is not the luxury of telling the patient that his or her problem is not well enough understood at this time and to come back later.

This process is well adapted to the fourth challenge of the ill-structured problem where the problem solver cannot be certain that a particular diagnosis or treatment plan is the correct one. The physician has to face ambiguities and insufficiency of needed data and make decisions on the basis of prevalence, probability, treating the treatable and watching out for the worst possibilities that could be present.

Metacognitive skills

This term refers to thinking about your own thinking. It is deliberation or pondering and is the very opposite of impulsivity. Metacognition is the hallmark of the expert: "Do I have the right ideas?" "What questions should I ask next?" "Can this problem be put together differently?" "Is there something I need to learn to understand this problem better?" "What would be the correct laboratory test to order here?" These are metacognitive thoughts. Metacognition is clearly seen in the expert when a patient problem is difficult or unusual. It is a skill the student should develop in guiding his or her own reasoning process. As mentioned before, this reasoning process of the physician is often not apparent to the physician as it is performed almost below awareness and often quickly and seemingly automatic. Only when physicians are confronted by a patient problem that is unusual, difficult or confusing are they aware of pondering the problem and actually considering alternative diagnostic ideas (hypotheses), questions that should be asked, items of physical examination that should be performed, laboratory tests that should be ordered (inquiry strategy), reviewing the findings obtained (analysis) or puzzling about what may be going on with the patient (synthesis). In fact, as mentioned before, experienced physicians may be so familiar with certain common, recurrent patient problems that they may take quick short cuts to establish and treat the problem. This has been called using heuristics, rules of thumb or forward reasoning. However, as also mentioned before, put an unfamiliar or troublesome problem in front of the experienced physician and you will see metacognition and the hypothetico-deductive process in full bloom.

The presence of the hypothetico-deductive process is usually not apparent to those watching physicians perform, as they do not know what is actually going on in the physician's mind. The observer can only guess as to the hypotheses being entertained by the questions being asked of the patient. Most physicians jump back and forth from a problem-oriented inquiry to a menu-driven inquiry as they are thinking, and the observer never knows which questions are hypothesis related. The observer also does not know how the data obtained are being analyzed. Techniques such as asking the physician to talk aloud during the patient encounter (usually with simulated patients), or to interview the physician about his or her thinking during an immediate videotaped replay of the patient encounter (stimulated recall) have been used in research on physician reasoning to analyze their reasoning.

The reasoning of scientists is no different than that of physicians. They also use the hypothetico-deductive method when faced with a problem or question.[39,40,41] One major difference is that it is next to impossible to rigorously rule out a hypothesis in medicine. The vagaries of disease expression and the differences in people, their response to disease and their ability to communicate prevent the physician from being confident that a remotely possible hypothesis is not actually present. In addition, the major objective of the physician is to care for the patient, as opposed to furthering the frontiers of science through detailed investigation of the patient's illness. The diagnoses entertained and the actions taken are often primarily for relief or symptomatic improvement. Lastly, as already mentioned, unlike many problems in science, decisions about diagnosis and treatment should be made despite inadequate and ambiguous data. A more detailed description of this reasoning process and how it can be developed can be found elsewhere.[30]

Reasoning pathologies

The hypothetico-deductive reasoning process could be assumed to be a natural process for anyone facing a problem in which more information is needed to understand and resolve the problem, as we have all been confronted with such problems all our lives. However, one cannot assume that this process is intact in the medical student. A number of "pathologies" can be seen in students using techniques such as stimulated recall, discussions around a simulated patient problem during a "time-in/time-out" period,[42] or computer simulations that track reasoning.[43] The following are some of the more commonly seen pathologies of the reasoning process in students and residents. These pathologies are not due to lack of knowledge, as the subjects can frequently recall the information that was not employed in the reasoning process when asked questions by the interviewer.

Anchoring

In this pathology, students generate an initial hypothesis about the patient's problem and then hang on to it throughout the encounter, despite information that surfaces in the encounter that weakens or even denies the likelihood of it being the correct hypothesis. Either the student deliberately does not look for information that would weaken an entertained hypothesis (as a good scientist would) or ignores such negative information when it appears.

Premature closure

This is a variation of anchoring. The student prematurely accepts a hypothesis as being the correct one when data obtained early in the encounter suggests it. The student fails to consider possible alternative hypotheses that could also be supported by the data obtained. Premature closure is usually triggered by a pathognomic symptom, sign, or a well-recognized syndrome. Perhaps the penchant many physicians have for looking for unlikely hypotheses or "rare birds" as possible diagnoses is used to prevent premature closure on an obvious, but possibly incorrect, hypothesis.

One hypothesis at a time

This is a very inefficient way to evaluate a patient. When only one hypothesis is entertained at a time, the student has to start over again when that particular hypothesis cannot be established resulting in an inefficient, laborious process. The risk of premature closure is also great.

No hypotheses

Incredibly, there are a number of students who seemingly do not generate any hypotheses at all or deliberately ignore any that come to mind, and depend on memorized lists of questions. Their workup of the patient is totally menu-driven with reviews of systems and other lists. Not only is this inefficient, it risks failing to make the correct diagnosis. When students do not know what it is they are looking for, they may not recognize important cues when they are in front of them and will not persist in ferreting out important information through alternative questions and examinations. This type of patient assessment with long lists of organ system reviews is often encouraged in early clinical courses (Physical Diagnosis, Introduction to Clinical Medicine) and in clerkships where students are rewarded more for asking all of the questions, as opposed to asking the right ones.

Incomplete set of hypotheses

The hypotheses generated by the student may lack important hypotheses that should always be considered with a particular presenting problem. The hypotheses generated may be too constricted or narrowed. When the set is incomplete and an important hypothesis that should be considered is missing, an incorrect diagnosis may be reached.

Disengaged inquiry

This is also a common problem among students. With this pathology, the student may generate a good set of hypotheses, but then does not carry out an inquiry strategy to deduce the most likely hypothesis. Instead, like the menu-driven students described previously, the student just asks a routine set of questions with every patient. After having spent a fair time interviewing and examining the patient, the student with disengaged inquiry usually fails to have a better idea of the probable diagnosis or differential diagnosis than existed at the start of the encounter.

Endless inquiry without decisions

Some students are not able to come to a conclusion about the patient's problem and continue to ask questions long after all the information needed to come to reasonable diagnostic or treatment conclusions has been obtained. They seem unable to make diagnostic decisions.

Forcing the diagnosis

Students often become enthusiastic about finding certain disease entities, especially ones they have just heard about and have caught their fancy. They attempt to find the disease in every patient. They tend to ask very direct, forcing and closed questions (reinforced with head nodding and voice emphasis) to get the patient to admit to the symptoms sought to establish the diagnosis. They will often overread or over-interpret questionable or equivocal patient responses and physical findings.

There are many other pathologies

These are only a few of the pathologies that can be seen in the reasoning process of medical students. Unfortunately, they can also be found in residents and physicians. They will not be recognized by either students or teachers unless appropriate tools are used to assess their reasoning. The existence of these pathologies underlines the importance of designing the educational process to help students acquire an accurate and efficient clinical reasoning process.

The hypothetico-deductive reasoning process is a complex skill. Like any complex skill (in science, music, sports, technical skills) it can only be developed through repeated practice with feedback. Teachers may agree that this process cannot be considered to be intact in the medical student but feel that the clinical clerkship is the appropriate place for students to develop reasoning skills. The case will be made in the next section that clinical reasoning skills should be practiced and used as the student is learning the basic science underpinnings to clinical practice from the first day of medical school, if the information learned is to be recalled and translated into care at the bedside when the clinical reasoning process is being employed.

Chapter Five

THE CLINICAL REASONING PROCESS IS ONLY PART OF THE PICTURE IN SOLVING THE PATIENT'S PROBLEM

Although the clinical reasoning process is an important vehicle for applying the physician's knowledge and expertise in a logical or scientific way to the solution of the patient's problem, it would be of no value without an extensive and rich medical knowledge base to support it. Both process and knowledge are required. A student with an extensive knowledge base, who might do well answering oral or written questions but who does not have good reasoning skills, will be ineffective as a physician. By contrast, good reasoning skills can help when knowledge is insufficient. It is impossible for any physician to have all the knowledge that will be needed for all patient problems that will be encountered. In fact, it is not uncommon for a patient to present a problem for which the physician does not have sufficient knowledge, but careful reasoning with the extensive knowledge that the physician does have can carry him or her quite far with the patient problem.

This relationship of content to process skills might be more clearly appreciated in an analogy with card playing. To be successful in a game of cards it certainly helps to have the right cards. However, having all the right cards may not help the poor player. In contrast, the expert player can usually do quite well with even poor cards. This is all summed up in a statement attributed to Herbert Simon that process and content are like the blades in a pair of scissors, they should work together to cut through a problem. We need to take a closer look at the relationship of knowledge to the physician's reasoning process.

The knowledge physicians bring to bear on the patient's problem is almost automatically recalled to mind with the cues presented by the patient's problem. More can be recalled through thoughtful deliberation (metacognition, as described previously in the clinical reasoning process). The recalled information is structured through associations with information from a variety of areas such as anatomy, physiology, pathology, psychology etc. and applied to the understanding of the patient problem as it unfolds. As only examples, the understanding of a patient with suspected gall-bladder disease depends on recall of anatomical, physiological, pathological, biochemical and pharmacological information associated around the evolving information on history, physical and laboratory tests. The assessment and treatment of a patient with suspected diabetic coma requires considerable biochemical and physiological knowledge. Often the experienced physician is unaware of the existence of knowledge itself, but its presence is clear in the tailored diagnostic and treatment decisions made on the unique picture a particular patient presents. Importantly, this rich, integrated and structured information base is enmeshed with the physician's clinical reasoning process. It is involved in the hypotheses generated through association with the cues in the patient's problem as well as in the inquiry, analysis, synthesis, and decision-making phases of the physician's reasoning. Most of these rich associations were acquired through prior patient experiences and learning related to those experiences.

The clinical reasoning process employed, and the associated information recalled and applied in work with the patient is not apparent to most practicing physicians as it is recalled and applied almost automatically and below consciousness. Only when deliberation or puzzlement intervenes and there is an active attempt to recall relevant information are physicians aware of their thinking and the information in memory.

Although much of the prior information learned in the context of work with similar patient problems will strongly influence the specific actions a physician may take on history, physical, laboratory test, and treatment of a patient problem, the physician may not be able to actually recall the reasons for the actions taken. Studies of patients with bilateral temporal lobe lesions who have no recent verbal memory have demonstrated that they can learn to problem solve as well as people with intact memories. They are able to apply what was learned to a problem months later, although they have no memory of the problem and deny ever seeing the problem previously or solving it. This suggests that memories that lead to actions, of knowing how to do something and memories describing things verbally may be in anatomically different systems.[44] This probably explains the expert's "knowing in action" described by Schon.[45] The physician shows expertise through actions, decisions and comments, but may not be able to describe the knowledge or facts basic to those actions. Unfortunately, for the reasons described above, physicians often tell students that much of what they had to learn in the basic sciences was not useful in clinical practice as they are not able to recall the basic science concepts behind their actions. This opinion, although incorrect, is understandable. Nevertheless, put any physician in front of a complex patient problem such as a severe electrolyte disturbance and you will see rich basic science information in action.

Figure 1 shows the recall of integrated basic science information, structured around the patient problem, and enmeshed with the clinical reasoning process in the mind of the physician. "A" could represent

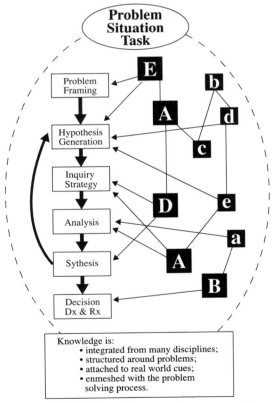

Fig.1 Relationship of content to the reasoning process of the patient

anatomical information, "B" biochemical information, "C" could be physiology, "D" could represent psychology etc. The capital letters represent major concepts and small letters represent minor concepts.

The structure of memory and its linkage to cognitive process in conventional educational approaches

As just discussed, the physician has information integrated from the sciences basic to medicine structured around the cues and information coming from the patient problem and enmeshed with the stages of the clinical reasoning process. Most was acquired during the clerkship, residency and practice, as much of the information acquired during conventionally taught basic science or preclinical years was forgotten. Levine and Forman presented 50 clinically relevant questions to students beginning their clerkship in neurology. These questions were taken from their final examination in the neuroscience course they had taken in the first year and passed. After attempting to answer those 50 questions, 62% of students had scores below the minimal pass level, and a number of scores were close to chance. The authors concluded that "a substantial number of students fail to retain the information taught in the preclinical years."[46]

In contrast to the integrated, patient-structured information that the physician has enmeshed with the clinical reasoning process, medical students in traditional preclinical years are asked to learn information from the basic sciences in isolated subject contexts, as shown in Figure 2. Even the so-called "integrated" basic science curricula in some schools still present information from the basic sciences in isolation from each other, but juxtaposed in the teaching schedule, usually in organ system units. Integration occurs in the schedule, not in the minds of the students. Information from each basic science discipline is learned in the context of that discipline and not in the context of patient problems. Concepts are learned within hierarchies of a particular discipline. The students in this traditional approach learn definitions and concepts in ways that will help them pass the written examinations they will get in subject contexts. The important cues for the recall of information acquired are the questions that will be on the examination, not cues that will appear with patient problems in later clinical work when the information will be needed to care for the patients. The principal cognitive skill students employ to survive in traditional curricula is rote memorization. This allows them to recall the information given in the course when asked for in examination questions that are aimed at the recall of content for its own sake. Information learned by rote memorization that is not actively applied or used will be quickly forgotten; not unlike the memorization of telephone numbers, addresses or nonsense syllables.

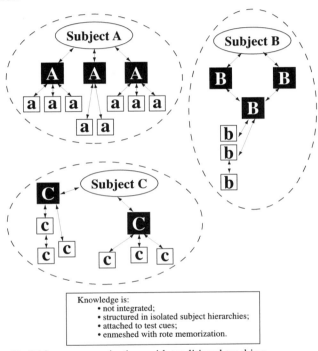

Fig.2 Memory organizations with traditional teaching

Student performance on an examination at the end of a basic science course does not measure long term recall or what they actually learned, as students will always cram to tune-up their long-term memory using rote memorization and mnemonics. Even if some basic science information were to be remembered by the time of the clinical years, it would not be associated with clinical phenomena (cues from the patient history, physical, and laboratory tests) or the clinical reasoning process employed. This severely reduces the odds that it will be recalled in subsequent clinical work.

Baddeley had one group of Royal Navy divers memorize a list of words under water and another group memorize a list on the land. He then divided each group in half and asked one half to recall the words in the environment where they were memorized and the other half to recall them in the environment where they did not memorize them. Those that had to recall them in the environment where they did not memorize them (those who memorized them on the shore recalling the words under water, and those who memorized them under water recalling them on the shore) could only recall two thirds as many words as those recalling them in the same environment.[47] Context is important in the recall of information. Thinking of those Royal Navy divers trying to recall information learned on the shore while under water is humorous, but not any more humorous than a student trying to recall information learned in a classroom while in the clinic.

The conventional method of learning basic science information is tragically inefficient when you take the long view beyond the final examination in the course. The students study very hard during their preclinical years to cram all that information into their heads and pass the course examinations. The faculty work very hard to put across the important facts and concepts in their disciplines, updating their offerings every year to be contemporary with changes in their field. Yet to what end? Much that was learned through all that effort will soon be forgotten, and what is remembered will not be recalled in the clinical contexts in which the student will be working. Problem-based learning addresses this inefficiency.

In order to "manage the health problems of patients in an effective, efficient and humane manner," the physician has to acquire an expert clinical reasoning process enmeshed with rich associated information structures that are recalled in the context of patient problems. Conventional basic science curricula do not stress the development of reasoning skills in the context of learning. The students are involved in passive learning in which their heads are force fed with "inert" knowledge as they try to absorb and memorize the great number of facts thrown at them in lectures and reading assignments. The term "inert knowledge" has been attributed to Alfred North Whitehead and is defined as knowledge that can be recalled to answer questions, but cannot be applied even though it is relevant, to the task at hand. Students' knowledge is acquired in the context of individual subjects and not integrated in the mind of the student around the pathophysiological, psychobiological or social problems of patients.

A study by Regan-Smith, Small, et al. questioned preclinical medical students from six medical schools about how they learned. One school was completely problem-based, two had traditional curricula, and three had both problem-based and traditional curricula. They compared the traditional students with the problem-based students. Their study showed that students in the preclinical years of a traditional curriculum devoted a large percentage of their learning to "memorization without understanding." The students in problem-based curricula devoted only a small percentage of their time to this activity and the difference was significant (p<.0001). The authors stated that the results "suggest that much education in traditional Year I and II curricula is useless for problem solving."[48]

Chapter Six

SELF-DIRECTED LEARNING

The second basic goal for undergraduate medical education as described in Chapter II is for students to develop the ability to "continue learning throughout their entire professional lives in order to meet the often unique and changing needs of patients and the problems they present, the changing problems and demands of the health care system, and to keep contemporary in medical knowledge and practice." The umbrella term for this ability is self-directed learning. Many physicians do not keep contemporary with their field and become outdated in their practice. A study of the hypertensive care provided by local physicians caring for members of a large group of steel workers indicated that the length of time since graduation from medical school correlated inversely with the quality of the care given by the physician.[49] Studies that examined the performance of practicing internists on a certifying examination a number of years after they had originally passed the examination suggested that there was "insufficient acquisition of new knowledge after training is completed." [50] The skill of self-directed learning has the following component skills.

Self-monitoring

Physicians should be able to continuously monitor their progress with a patients' problems noting where they may be puzzled or lack the appropriate knowledge or skills. Self-monitoring requires a deliberate attempt to be aware of how well different aspects of each patient's problem are being handled, the accuracy of the diagnosis, or the appropriateness of the management undertaken. Was there a problem in generating appropriate hypotheses or in inquiring against the hypotheses that were considered? Were the history questions, items of the physical examination, or laboratory tests the most appropriate? How much confidence was used to make the diagnosis(es) and select the treatment plan? Is there a better one? What needs to be researched? etc.

Self-assessment

In addition to monitoring their performance, physicians should be able to determine if their performance is appropriate for the type of patient problems they are encountering. It is too easy just to do what you have always done or to refer the patient to someone else and go on to the next patient without considering whether the care of the patient should have been better. Of great concern are physicians who are not aware of inadequacies in their work with patients and do not refer or ask for help.

Defining learning needs

Once inadequacies or weaknesses are recognized in practice, they should be translated into clearly defined learning needs so that the appropriate or most effective learning resource can be identified. What specific areas of information and or skills are needed?

Determining the appropriate learning resource

Physicians should be able to determine what available learning resource would be the most effective and practical for their defined learning need. Where can they get up-to-date and accurate information (personal textbooks, monographs or reviews, journal articles, computerized, online information resources, library resources, videotapes, videodiscs, friends, consultants, continuing medical education course, etc).

Using the resource effectively

It is one thing to select the right resource and another to use the resource effectively. This is particularly true with computerized or online information resources.

Evaluating the accuracy and value of the information in the resource

It is important for physicians to question the findings or opinions of a consultant or author and compare them with other information and opinions. The methods used in a research report, the data obtained, and the validity of conclusions drawn should be evaluated by the physician. This is increasingly important with the availability of computer databases that, unlike those in the library, are often not reviewed or refereed. It is this important skill that is being emphasized in evidence-based medicine.[51]

Recording or filing the information for future reference

Once information has been obtained, physicians should have a systematic way to file it for future reference where it can be conveniently found when needed again.

Applying what has been learned to the present patient problem and future problems

To close the self-study chain of activities, physicians should then apply what has been learned back to the care of their patients.

Physicians have to assume responsibility for their continued learning following completion of their formal education. In order to be able do this effectively, the required skills need to be developed and practiced while they are in medical school under faculty guidance and assistance. Self-directed learning should become a reflex habit for physicians so that they will, without effort or thought, keep contemporary in their practice and to meet the changing problems presented by patients and the many changes in their particular field.

The skills required in the clinical reasoning process and the skills required for self-directed learning need to be practiced again and again by medical students under the guidance of faculty teachers and with feedback from peers and tutors to achieve the effectiveness expected of today's physicians.

For knowledge acquired in medical school to be recalled and applied to the care of patients, these skills should be acquired in the context of work with patient problems from the first day of medical school. That is the context in which the skills and information will be needed and recalled by the student as physician.

Chapter Seven

THE EDUCATIONAL OBJECTIVES THAT ARE ADDRESSED BY AUTHENTIC PROBLEM-BASED LEARNING

The discussions in the preceding chapters set the stage for a consideration of the educational objectives that serve as a guide to the appropriate design of the problem-based learning experience.

Problem-based learning asks students to learn by working in the context of medical problems, those of individual patients and communities of patients. The problems are presented to the students in formats that allow students to apply the same clinical reasoning skills that are required in clinical practice. In doing this, the students discover what information needs to be learned from the sciences basic to medicine to fully understand the patient problem, the mechanisms responsible for the problem (down to the organ, tissue, cellular or molecular level as appropriate), and the normal structure and functions of the systems and structures involved. The information acquired is integrated from many disciplines and structured around the context of patient problems. In authentic problem-based learning, students learn to become responsible for their own learning, defining what needs to be learned in their problem work and the appropriate resources to use (faculty, consultants, books, monographs, journal articles, automated information sources, etc.). They apply what they have learned to the problem at hand and to future problems.

Putting all of this together, this educational method addresses the following educational objectives for the medical student:

1) The acquisition of an extensive knowledge base that is:
   a) Integrated from multiple discipline/subject areas
   b) Retained in long term memory
   c) Structured for application to patient problems
   d) Recalled in association with patient problem cues that occur in clinical contexts
   e) Enmeshed with the clinical reasoning process used in clinical practice.

2) The development of
   a) Clinical reasoning skills that are effective and efficient
   b) Independent, self-directed learning skills that are
      effective, efficient, and habitual
   c) Skills in history taking, physical examination, patient
      education, communication and interpersonal skills
   d) The ability to work effectively in a team setting by working
      collaboratively, assisting peers in their learning, learning from
      peers, and accepting and giving constructive feedback
   e) An internal motivation to learn, question, and understand

3) An early and continued immersion into the culture and values of
   medicine as a profession to become aware of such things as:
   a) The ambiguities of practice and the limits of knowledge
   b) The fact that experts can hold differing opinions
   c) The responsibilities and obligations of the physician in caring
      for individual patients and communities of patients
   d) The moral and ethical dilemmas of medicine
   e) The complexities of health care delivery and the financial bur-
      dens and inequities involved

Whether any or all of these are successfully addressed in any variety
of problem-based learning depends on the design of the particular
problem-based learning method. They are all addressed in authentic
problem-based learning.

The many varieties of problem-based learning

The differences between authentic problem-based learning methods
and many other problem-based learning methods can be best understood in terms of these objectives. For example, if the development
of effective, efficient skills in clinical reasoning is not thought to be
necessary or a concern for the preclinical years, the problems used
will not be designed to present students with an ill-structured problem in which free inquiry is possible, and tutors will not be trained
to help the students develop their reasoning skills. Instead, the
patient problem will be used primarily as a signpost to indicate what
information needs to be acquired in considering the various things
that could be wrong with the patient. This situation occurs in many

schools employing problem-based learning. If the acquisition of integrated basic science information structured around patient problems is not thought of as an important concern or objective, then lecture courses in various disciplines may precede or accompany the student's problem-based learning experiences. If self-directed learning is not considered an important objective for medical students, the problem-based learning method employed will not be designed in a manner that encourages and helps students to develop these skills, and the students will not have the time and opportunity to carry it out. Instead, the faculty will prescribe what should be learned after the students have encountered the problem and the resources to be used. Ignoring this objective makes problem-based learning teacher-centered, and students are denied the privilege of taking the responsibility for their own learning, becoming independent thinkers and enjoying working on their own. The importance of student-centered learning has to be fully understood by all the faculty involved in problem-based learning, particularly the tutors, to ensure that it is truly student-centered. It is almost a reflex for medical school teachers to want to give information to students and to suggest to students what they ought to learn, even when they know its the wrong thing to do. One school with a problem-based learning curriculum that describes self-directed learning as a goal nevertheless provided their students with suggested topics for study and prescribed references during their work with the problem. Another allowed resource faculty to give the students presentations on what they felt the students should know about the problem they were studying. Still others give students written examinations that suggest to the students that there is a prescribed content to be learned. Tutors who do not understand problem-based learning or who have been inadequately trained can direct student's thinking in many subtle ways.

In some schools with problem-based learning there are disciplines that are not included and are taught separately in a more conventional manner in some schools. Anatomy and biochemistry, for example, are taught outside of an existing problem-based curriculum.

The perceived time, expense and trouble involved in pursuing certain of these objectives in problem-based learning may be a factor in these things not being incorporated into the design of the curriculum. This is particularly true in the design of problems. To design and author written or printed problems in a way that will present the patient problem as it actually occurred in practice, as an ill-structured problem, and to allow for free inquiry on history, physical and laboratory tests takes more time than writing a case report. Several schools with a problem-based learning curriculum have identified this as the principal reason for using complete, or well-structured, case reports.

Many of these objectives such as the development of the clinical reasoning process and self-directed study skills require an understanding of these skills on the part of the tutor, which in turn requires tutor training.

Despite these wide variations, most schools that claim to have a problem-based learning curriculum use problems as a central stimulus for learning, and learning is usually in small groups with a teacher in the role of a tutor. Beyond that, as suggested above, there is great latitude. Problem-based learning has been very liberally interpreted by some faculty to include any use of any kind of problem at some time somewhere in the context of an ongoing lecture series or laboratory course.[52] When reading about a problem-based learning method or hearing a presentation about a problem-based learning method, it is important to learn exactly how it is delivered, the design of the problem used, the degree to which it is student-centered, the process used in the tutorial group, is it given within a single discipline or are disciplines integrated, and how students are evaluated among other things. This is discussed in more detail in Chapter XIV.

As a particular species of problem-based learning, authentic problem-based learning is designed to address all of the objectives described above. Problems are ill-structured. Students can inquire freely as in the real clinical situation, and self-directed learning is required, as students become increasingly responsible for their own learning. Learning is integrated from all disciplines in the basic sciences, and assessment is designed to assess the students ability to apply knowledge using reasoning and self-directed study skills, and students are assessed for their progress towards these objectives.

Chapter Eight

THE CURRICULAR REQUIREMENTS OF AUTHENTIC PROBLEM-BASED LEARNING

This chapter describes the things that are required to mount an authentic problem-based learning curriculum in the preclinical or basic science years, for either an alternative, parallel track or for the entire class.

Tutors

The tutor has the responsibility of facilitating student learning in the small group. The role of the tutor is not unlike an athletic, dance, or musical tutor who encourages excellence in performance through active guidance from the sidelines. Tutors can be from the clinical or basic science faculty. They can be nurses, residents, psychologists, social workers, educators, senior medical students or graduate students. In the second preclinical year, physicians may be important as they can provide a role model for students about to enter their clinical years and can underline the clinical relevance of the students' learning.

Tutors should receive training for their role! The success or failure of a problem-based learning curriculum can rest on the preparation and training of tutors, as their skills are central to the delivery of the curriculum. The universal experience of all PBL curricula is that the skill and understanding of the tutor is essential to success. This role is central to the students' abilities to achieve the educational goals possible with authentic problem-based learning. The skillful tutor will encourage the students to develop effective reasoning skills, acquire a solid knowledge base, become effective self-directed learners, take control of their own learning, and enjoy the whole process. The skillful tutor will also be able to eventually fade away and allow the students to carry on the process by themselves.

Recurrent tutorial workshops are necessary for all new faculty and to polish and further perfect the skills of those who have been tutors. These workshops should truly be workshops and require the participant to practice working in the tutorial role under the supervision of an experienced tutor. Videotaping tutorial sessions with feedback is also a valuable adjunct to training. Some schools have also found it valuable to have a new tutor candidate sit in with an experienced tutor.

The ideal small group size is 5 to 7 students. Below that number, the amount of pooled knowledge the group can bring to the problem and the value of different points of view and approaches to a problem is seriously reduced. If the group is larger than 7 students, it becomes difficult for the tutor to keep track of all students and for all students to have a chance to express their particular points of view in the various stages of work with the problem, and the group's working sessions become longer to allow for each student's ideas and comments in all discussions.

At the end of each curricular unit, usually 8 to 10 weeks, the tutor is changed and the students are randomly reassembled into new groups. This is important to encourage the development of team skills, as students have to learn to work with a changing variety of people. In a new unit the students and tutor are all new to each other.

Tutors usually have to plan on spending around 6 to 9 hours a week for the 8 to 10 weeks of a problem-based learning curricular unit (2 to 3 hour sessions). It is usually too demanding for tutors to take on two groups in a curriculum unit unless they are able to set aside 25 to 30% of their time for tutoring during the unit. Even experienced tutors find two groups more effort than they anticipated.

There has been much discussion over the years as to whether tutors need to be expert in the subject area in which they are tutoring. There is little question that the best combination is for a well-trained tutor to also be an expert in the particular content area in which the group is studying. Students' learning can be facilitated in ways that minimize students going down unproductive pathways. Of course it is valuable for students to go down wrong pathways and discover during self-directed learning the folly of their ways. However the effective expert tutor will allow this to happen as well, but will also be sure that the students maximize on their experience, without loss of the experience being student-centered. If a curriculum is to be limited to using expert tutors, as opposed to using all available faculty, clinical and basic science as well as residents and senior students, then the numbers available is limited. If you are not able to provide enough well-trained, experienced tutors who are expert in the area of a unit, you are forced to choose between tutors who are well-trained and effective as tutors, but not expert, versus tutors who are not effective or well trained as tutors but experts. There is little question but that the latter is undesirable, as the skills of the tutor are fundamental to the effectiveness of problem-based learning. Tutors are not expected to dispense information; content learning in the area of the unit occurs during self-directed study. It is at this time that students can work with resource faculty who are expert in the area of their specific learning issues.

The practice at Southern Illinois University is to make certain all tutors have attended a workshop on tutoring, and while they are tutoring they are asked to meet once a week to discuss tutoring problems that may have been encountered. In addition, all tutors in a particular unit are provided with an orientation to the unit and information about each problem, why it is being used in the unit and expected learning objectives that might be accomplished by their group with the problem. This helps non-expert tutors gain the degree of the expertise needed to be comfortable in their role. The expectations of the tutor as a coach in the development of clinical reasoning and self-directed learning and as a guide to the structure of the problem-based learning sequences are quite specific. And the role of the tutor is not passive; it is a very active one. (See the companion volume to this book, *The Tutorial Process*, concerning the role of the tutor and the skills involved.[1])

Resource faculty (consultants)

These are faculty teachers who have agreed to be available to students during their self-directed study. They are a source for references and for information from their particular area of expertise (basic science or clinical field). A better term for resource faculty is "consultant" as the students are using them as consultants and developing the skills needed to work with consultants in the future.

Discussions with resource faculty are arranged by the students and can be with one or more students or a discussion with the entire small group. Sometimes several groups all identify the need for information from a resource faculty and ask for a lecture to be given to the entire problem-based learning class. Such a lecture requested by the students is most appropriate as it represents student-centered and student-initiated learning. In any discussions with a resource faculty, it is expected that students will have already carried out their own preliminary study in the areas of their questions. Resource faculty should question students that have come to them about what they have looked up prior to the consultation, and to ask them enough questions about the topic to see what they already know so that the information given can be tailored to their needs. If resource faculty find that the students have not done enough prior study, they can suggest references that ought to be read before talking to them.

Each resource faculty indicates the times during the week that they are available to consult with students and how they can be contacted. Some resource faculty may also spend as much as 6 to 9 hours a week during one unit of 8 to 10 weeks and may only be listed during one unit in a year. It is best if they plan on doing interruptible work during their available hours as a resource, so that they get work done if no students show up.

Sometimes resource faculty finds that they are constantly being contacted about the same subject by different groups of students. This can be alleviated if the resource faculty puts together a learning resource that covers that subject for the students to study first, and then come back later if there are unanswered questions.

Problem simulations

All the problem simulations used in authentic problem-based learning are based on actual patient cases. The findings on history and physical examination as well as the laboratory results, x-rays, imaging, electrocardiograms, etc. of the patient are incorporated into the simulation for the students to use in their work with the patient's problem. In problem-based learning, the problems present themselves to the students in the same way and with the same information that was available in the real clinical situation. All simulation formats are designed to allow the students to ask the patient any question, perform any item of physical examination, order any laboratory or diagnostic procedure they feel appropriate in any order - just as in the real clinical situation. At no place in any simulation should the student be told that a question is inappropriate or was never asked in the real situation or that no information is available. The students will, of course, ask questions, perform items of physical examination and order tests that were never carried out on the actual patient. The physician who cared for the actual patient, on whom the case is based, authors the simulations used in problem-based learning. He uses creative authorship and knowledge of the patient and the disease process involved to make available all the answers that could be obtained on history, all the results on physical examination and laboratory results that would be found had those items of inquiry actually been performed on the patient. Therefore, as in the real clinical situation, students are able to ask inappropriate questions and perform inappropriate examinations or tests and get the responses that would occur with the actual patient. This ensures that the simulations used, as in the PBLMs (described below), present the ill-structured problems that real patients present and with free inquiry provide the same challenge to clinical reasoning as the actual patient.

Problem-based learning modules (PBLMs)

These are simulations bound and printed in book form that meet the above requirements for patient problem simulations.[27] Based on actual patients, the PBLM presents the patient problem exactly as it presented clinically with only the initial information available, usually the chief complaint and the health care setting in which the patient is encountered. They are designed so anything that can be done with the actual patient in the way of history and physical examination can be carried out with the PBLM. All questions on history and items of the physical examination can be performed in any sequence, and the student learns immediately the patient's answer or the finding on physical examination. At no time should the student get an answer of "inappropriate" or "not done" for any question or examination even if irrelevant to the patient's problem or inappropriate-as is true in real life. Also true to real life, such comments as "normal" or "no findings" cannot be found, just the data that would be obtained from the action taken with the patient.

Laboratory tests can also be ordered and the results can be learned at the time or with an appropriate delay for the test, depending on the educational goals of the group while working with the PBLM. In addition, the PBLM allows the patient's problem to be followed over time, and the students can see how the actual case was managed by those caring for the patient. In addition to the patient's answers and questions, findings on examination and laboratory and diagnostic tests, the PBLM contains these additional materials that provide feedback to the student about their performance with the problem:

1) Learning issues that should be generated by the student group in the opinion of faculty from a variety of disciplines. These are referred to by the students only after they have completed their work with the problem, including all self-directed study. It serves as a guide to the students in subsequent self-directed study and is not intended to be a prescription. (This list can also be given to the tutor as a guide to issues that the students might profitably identify. The tutor shares the list with the group after they have finished with the PBLM.)

2) A data sheet that contains all the important elements in the problem as a guide to faculty in their selection and use of the problem that is not looked at by the students.

3) The relative costs of all laboratory and diagnostic tests.

4) A patient follow-up section. After the students have decided on their diagnosis and treatment of the patient, they can follow the diagnosis and treatment given by those who had cared for the patient and subsequent
clinical course of the patient.

A booklet called the "User's Guide" that accompanies all PBLMs lists all the actions possible on history and physical as well as laboratory tests and diagnostic procedures so that students can readily lookup the patient's response to their actions in the PBLM. The guide also suggests various ways the PBLM can be used in different educational settings and with varying educational goals.

Standardized (simulated) patients

Standardized patients are people trained to present an actual patient's problem in a manner so convincing that a clinician cannot differentiate them from actual patients.[42] They can be interviewed and examined as the actual patient. The standardized patient allows students to also learn and practice history and physical examination skills, communication and interpersonal skills as they work through the problem. Standardized patients are trained to always present a patient problem in a real and consistent manner.

The so-called "time-in, time-out" technique allows the standardized patient to be used for clinical teaching in the small group format. One student takes on the role of the physician or examiner and begins the patient interview. Whenever the students or the tutor wish to discuss what is going on in the patient problem and to discuss student thinking about the problem at the moment, a "time-out" is declared. At this time the standardized patient remains in role as far as appearances go but will not respond to any questions while the interviewer presents his or her thinking and the rest of the group discusses their thinking about the case under the guidance of the tutor. The standardized patient's subsequent performance will continue unchanged or unaffected by any comments made as if the time out period and discussion had never occurred. When "time-in" is declared, the standardized patient continues on as though no time had passed since the "time-out." Once the simulated encounter is finished, the standardized patient can provide students feedback about their interpersonal and professional skills.

Simulated patients are trained to present the patient's problem in all of the PBLMs in which it is possible (the only limitation is whether the physical findings can be simulated). In some instances actual patients with stable findings who agree to working with students are used. This allows the small group to encounter the patient as either a PBLM or a living, breathing patient. If they start with the standardized patient, they can then continue with the PBLM using the database that they acquired from the standardized patient, order laboratory tests and follow the patient's course. This gives the small group flexibility in the objectives they wish to address.

Patients

From the very start of the problem-based learning curriculum, at least a half day every week should be set aside for students to work in clinical settings with patients to transfer what they have learned in their ongoing work with problem simulations to encounters with real patients. This cements the applicability of what they have learned to clinical work and extends their patient problem experience. They should be assigned to a physician who helps them with their clinical skills and arranges the patient contacts for them. It is important that the students have direct, active experience working with patients in these settings and are not just watching physicians at work. Attempts should be made to have the patients they encounter correlate with their ongoing work in the curriculum. If, for example, the students were in a cardio-respiratory unit, experience with cardiac and respiratory patients would be desirable. This clinical time can be further enhanced by assigning each student to the same clinician for an extended period of time, so that the clinician can help them acquire the fundamentals of history and physical examination and can provide them with increasing independence with patients as they progress. The clinicians are encouraged (trained, if possible) to use facilitatory teaching skills similar to that of the tutors.

Discipline consultants

Each basic science and clinical department is asked to identify a member of its faculty who will review the problems developed in the problem-based curriculum to see if, in their opinion, their discipline is being adequately covered. These consultants may suggest changes in some of the problems that might bring out certain learning issues or they might suggest other problems that may be needed. Besides being departmental representatives, other discipline consultants can represent other areas that need to be continuously addressed in the curriculum, such as, epidemiology, statistics and measurement, nutrition, geriatrics, ethics, legal matters, womens' issues, psychosocial concerns, etc. to ensure these areas are covered adequately with the problems used in the curriculum. This review is recurrent to keep the curriculum contemporary with changes in every field.

Home rooms

Each small group should have its own room for tutorial meetings, discussion and for study. This room provides the students a base for their work and a place where they can work individually or in groups whenever they wish 24 hours a day. These rooms should be locked and keys are available only to the members of the group, including the tutor. It is a room where the students can safely bring personal belongings, books, notes, charts, work materials, microscopes, or whatever. The rooms should have a table large enough for the students and the tutor as it serves as a meeting place for the small group and tutor to work through the problems in the unit and for the students to work and study. There should be a large chalk/feltpen board, x-ray viewbox, computer (with online capability to library and Internet) and storage space for books, specimens, and a variety of learning materials.

Learning resources

In authentic problem-based learning the students determine what it is they will need to learn as they work through the patient problem. The challenge of the problem and the stated objectives of the curricular unit, coupled with the students' awareness of their own knowledge deficiencies helps them decide what they need to learn. The medical library and the medical faculty are major resources. As no textbooks are prescribed in problem-based learning, the students are free to use whatever texts they find most helpful. Extra copies of texts and monographs that might be commonly used by the students in any particular unit can be put in the library. The print resources of the library are enhanced by computer-based information sources such as Medline and the Internet. Librarians should be prepared to assist students with information searches so that they can learn the most effective and efficient ways to get up-to-date and accurate information from the library.

Anatomical resources should also be available. Prosected cadavers, cadavers available for dissection, plastic embedded specimens, slide collections, plastic models, and the like, allow students to learn the anatomy involved in the patient problem first hand. Cadavers should also be available for students to dissect on their own, guided by anatomy faculty as consultants, if they are so stimulated in their ongoing problem work.

Pathology resources should also be available in slide sets, videodiscs, embedded specimens and the like. They are enhanced by necropsy experiences that correlate with the problems being studied.

Schedules

There should be no curricular schedules in problem-based learning except for:

1) The time of the initial orientation for students and tutors to a new unit

2) Weekly unit meetings of students and tutors to pass on announcements and to deal with concerns and complaints

3) Weekly clinical experiences

4) Examinations

Outside of that, scheduling should be left to each small group to work out on their own for the following reasons:

> The challenge of each problem varies with the background knowledge of the students in the group and their particular interests. Depending on where they are in a particular unit, a problem may require a number of tutorial sessions to complete especially the first problems in a unit. Other problems, later on, may require only one or two tutorial sessions as knowledge accumulates in the area of the unit and learning issues decrease in number.

> The tutorial sessions may vary in length depending on the discussions, ramifications of the problem, background and interests of the students, and the issues developed in the group.

> The type, number and complexity of the learning issues that each group identifies can vary widely.

> It may take a day or two for the students to obtain and use all the learning resources required for a problem. With another it may take only a few hours.

Some learning issues may require more time to accomplish depending on the availability of resource faculty or distances involved in obtaining information (such as a visit to an outside expert, a laboratory, clinic or other facility)

Most importantly, flexibility in the group's schedule allows each tutor to schedule the group meetings around his or her research, clinical or administrative activities. Groups can meet in the early morning or evenings or whenever it works out best for all the members of the group. This flexibility makes it easier for busy faculty to be educational tutors.

Each group should be able to schedule their own time for small group meetings throughout each week.

Even the weekly clinical experience can be scheduled by the group if they have an assigned clinical tutor to work with them.

Chapter Nine

THE AUTHENTIC PROBLEM-BASED LEARNING PROCESS

This chapter describes the sequence of activities the small group of students and tutor go through with each problem. This process is designed to address the educational objectives described previously in Chapter VII.

1) The acquisition of an extensive knowledge base that is:
   a) Integrated from multiple discipline/subject areas
   b) Retained in long term memory
   c) Structured for application to patient problems
   d) Recalled in association with patient problem cues that occur in clinical contexts
   e) Enmeshed with the clinical reasoning process used in clinical practice.

2) The development of
   a) Clinical reasoning skills that are effective and efficient
   b) Independent, self-directed learning skills that are effective, efficient, and habitual
   c) Skills in history taking, physical examination, patient education, communication and interpersonal skills
   d) The ability to work effectively in a team setting by working collaboratively, assisting peers in their learning, learning from peers, and accepting and giving constructive feedback
   e) An internal motivation to learn, question, and understand

3) An early and continued immersion into the culture and values of medicine as a profession to become aware of such things as:
   a) The ambiguities of practice and the limits of knowledge
   b) The fact that experts can hold differing opinions
   c) The responsibilities and obligations of the physician in caring for individual patients and communities of patients
   d) The moral and ethical dilemmas of medicine
   e) The complexities of health care delivery and the financial burdens and inequities involved.

Keep these objectives in mind as you read through the following sequence of activities employed in problem-based learning, and note where they are addressed.

When the small group first meets

At the start of each new curricular unit, the students are randomly assigned to groups and to a tutor. It is likely that many students in the group have not worked together before and do not know each other very well, even if they have been in the curriculum a while. These initial activities are designed to allow the group to know each other, to get comfortable talking to each other and to set the stage for the group working as a team.

Introductions

Students are asked to introduce themselves to the others in the group and describe the college or university attended prior to medical school, majors or studies undertaken and other activities that would be of interest. They might also describe their reasons for coming to medical school, anticipated career, hobbies and other interests.

This activity gives each member the opportunity to be recognized as an individual with an interesting and unique background. The members of the group find areas of common background and interests, facilitating communication and teamwork in the group. It allows each member of the group and the tutor to identify where particular experiences or expertise might provide a resource to the group.

This is information about students that faculty rarely learn in conventional curricula. Tutors are often amazed to discover the extensive education and experiences many students had before coming to medical school.

Tutors should also provide the students with their own background information.

Climate and roles

The learning climate in problem-based learning is quite different from that in conventional education and should be discussed. In much of conventional medical education, students learn to remain quiet if they are not confident of their knowledge and hope not to be chosen to comment. If they are asked to speak, they learn to bluff as well as possible, to avoid getting marked down for not knowing. This is counterproductive if we want students to be aware of what they know and what they need to learn. In problem-based learning, students should describe what they know, what they think they know and readily admit what they are unsure of in the group's ongoing discussions. This is basic to their realizing what they need to learn. New knowledge acquired in medical school should never be built on old misinformation. Students won't know if what they think is right unless they verbalize it and test it out in the group. If students hold back from speaking because they are not sure they are right, they may avoid providing a valuable insight or contribution. The tutor has to set the stage by making it clear that members of the group should say whatever is in their minds and freely admit when they don't know.

There also needs to be a climate of free and open exchange of opinions and points of view. The tutor stresses the need for members of the group to speak up when they disagree with what is being said by someone else, have a different point of view or opinion to offer, or do not understand what has been said. This includes what the tutor says. The rule should be established that if everyone remains silent after a contribution by a member of the group, that means that no one has a different opinion, information or idea and all agree with what is being said. In problem-based learning discussions, silence is assent.

It is one thing to say these things and another to be sure they are carried out in the group. The tutor should be certain that all opinions and comments are respected by the members of the group. The tutor should also be sure that all points of view and information are heard and that no one dominates the group's opinions or ideas. And above all, tutors should admit their own ignorance, confusion, or insecurity as a model for the students. In all aspects of small group process, the tutor should be a model for the behaviors and attitudes expected from the group.

Tutors should review the students' role and responsibilities and their own role and responsibility in the group. The tutor's role is to guide students through the problem-solving process and self-directed learning processes with leading questions and by challenging their thinking. The tutor will frequently ask students to explain or clarify their ideas and comments. The tutor will challenge students with "why" again and again, regardless of whether the tutor personally feels that a particular student's comment is right or wrong, in order to reveal the students' degree of understanding and ability to support or define what they are saying. This helps students understand what they know and what they need to learn. In this process, the tutors will do everything possible to keep the students from knowing their personal opinion. The tutor should not provide information to the group about any aspect of the problem, even though she or he might be an expert in an area under discussion. The students have to dig out information on their own from other sources than the tutor. Initially the tutor will spend considerable time guiding students in the problem-based and self-directed learning process until they get the hang of it.

As time goes on, students should assume more and more of the responsibility of managing the group's direction and process. The patient problem is their problem and they should take on the responsibility for problem solving and self-directed study. Students should challenge each other in the group discussions. They should also note this when they feel that the group process is going in the wrong directions or that there are interpersonal problems or conflicts developing in the group. The tutor should eventually become unnecessary in the successful problem-based learning group.

As the students gain in confidence about how to reason through a problem, identify learning needs, challenge each others ideas, discuss what they have learned, evaluate themselves and thereby gradually take on responsibility for the group process, the tutor will withdraw and play a smaller and smaller role. Refer to *The Tutorial Process* designed as a companion to this book for more detailed information on the tutor's role.[1]

The first session with a new problem

The problem is taken on by the group without prior preparation, even in the beginning of the first year or in a new curricular unit. This may be difficult for faculty and students used to conventional educational approaches to accept. Teachers often express the concern that the students do not have sufficient knowledge to begin problem solving with patient problems. They think the students would do far better if first they were to learn anatomy, physiology, biochemistry, etc. There is a tendency even for faculty involved in designing problem-based learning curricula to want to provide lectures and assign readings for a period of time before work with the patient problem begins. However, as reassuring as such prior preparation might be, there are a number of reasons why this is neither appropriate nor effective in problem-based learning. Taking on the problem as an unknown, without prior preparation, allows the students to discover what they already know or understand about the problem. We all have information in our heads that may only be recalled in certain contexts and by certain associations. For example, if a teacher were to be asked to give a talk on a particular subject in an area of expertise the next day, you can be sure that she or he would review textbooks, prior notes, or whatever. This is because it is so difficult to recall to mind all that you may know about a subject in the abstract. However, if that teacher were to be presented with a series of patients or research problems in her area of expertise, the needed information would flow into mind in association with the cues present by the problems and with the thinking used. The same is true of medical students. They have little appreciation of what they may already know from their prior education or prior experiences laid down in their long-term memory. The stimulus of a patient problem will often bring to mind information that may actually be a surprise to them. It is often a surprise for faculty as well to see how much information can be brought to bear on a patient problem even by first week medical students. Students are not tabula razas and have accumulated much knowledge in college, life experiences, reading, television etc. This ability of problem-solving work to bring forth prior knowledge has many advantages for learning. It indicates areas of information that may not need to be pursued in any great depth during self-directed study related to the patient problem. The knowledge pulled forth from memory during the encounter with the problem provides an anchor for remembering new knowledge acquired during study, ensuring better retention and recall. Also, the activated knowledge already in long-term memory can enhance the understanding of the related new knowledge acquired through self-study.

Of most importance, however, taking on the problem as an unknown without prior preparation allows students to realize what they need to learn to understand and resolve the problem. This is a motivating stimulus for learning. Students are puzzled and challenged by the problem and want to get the information needed to understand it. Motivation is further enhanced by the realization that this is the kind of problem they will have to face as physicians. The learning required to understand the problem is obviously relevant and important to their career.

If the integration of knowledge from different disciplines, structured around the cues presented by a patient problem and enmeshed with clinical reasoning is an important objective, then providing students with information during an initial period of learning unassociated with the problem or problem contexts is illogical and unproductive.

The last and perhaps most compelling reason for encountering the problem first without prior information or study is that this is the way the students will have to function as physicians in clinical practice. The patient always comes as an unknown and physicians will have to work as far as possible with the problem on the basis of knowledge already possessed. Never will the nurse tell them, for example, that there is a case of Italian Somaliland Camel-bite Fever in the waiting room and that they might look it up in a textbook before seeing the patient.

Objectives

When any group sits down to work in problem-based learning, it is essential that they agree on the task they are to undertake; what will be their learning objectives? A discussion of objectives focuses the group's tasks they will undertake with the patient problem. Any patient problem could raise a wide range of learning issues all the way from disorders at the molecular level through clinical symptoms and signs, epidemiology, treatment and issues of health care delivery. Problems will involve learning issues in most every discipline in the basic sciences, epidemiology, medical humanities, clinical sciences, the social sciences, etc. Conceivably, one problem could provide a yearlong curriculum. Therefore, it is important that the small group focuses on the specific learning objectives they would like to accomplish with the problem. If the problem-based learning curriculum is implemented as it usually is in the preclinical years, the tutor and the group need to agree that their problem-related learning should concentrate on the basic sciences; analyzing the mechanisms underlying the patient's problem. It is all too easy for medical students, as future physicians, to become engrossed with the clinical aspects of the problem and want to make a clinical diagnosis. A criticism often leveled at problem-based learning is that it allows medical students to play doctor prematurely and they do not acquire a solid foundation in the basic sciences. Agreeing that learning the basic science relevant to the problem is a major objective helps focus their learning to the appropriate depth of understanding for the basic sciences.

The group can also extend or modify their objectives based on areas of learning they are concerned about. These might be areas that have not been well covered with prior problems or areas of personal interest. A problem-based learning curriculum in the clinical years can focus on diagnosis, treatment, interpersonal skills, epidemiology, ethical and health care issues, etc.

A printed set of objectives for every curricular unit helps the group focus and agree upon the appropriate objectives. In the Appendix there is a sample set of objectives for a unit on the nervous system, musculoskeletal system and psychiatry that emphasizes basic science learning.

In this discussion of objectives, the tutor gets the group to agree on their objectives for the problem, and what it is they expect to accomplish in their learning at this time in the curriculum. This sets the focus for the discussions in the group. If they agree on learning in the basic science, then their problem solving, the hypotheses raised, the understanding of the problem that is developed, the learning issues agreed upon, and the group's self-evaluation will be guided by those agreed upon objectives. In accepting basic science learning, the group should understand that it means going deeper than the "black box" level (superficial explanations for concepts and observed phenomena) and going down to the tissue, cellular, or molecular level as appropriate in their learning issues and study.

When the group agrees that basic science learning is one of their learning objectives it becomes easier for the tutor to probe their thoughts and challenge them with "why" again and again. This forces students to get down to the basic mechanisms for the patient's problem.

When the group becomes immersed in a problem, they often get carried away by the many interesting things that develop, and interests and concerns surface that are peripheral to their agreed upon goals. As mentioned before, they will often become concerned about the clinical diagnosis, prognosis, and treatment. With an emergency problem they may totally forget their basic science focus and become concerned about the immediate care of the patient. When this happens, and it is recognized by the tutor (or preferably by the students), the agreed upon objectives can be used as a reference point for rethinking the direction of their discussions and learning. Sometimes it's appropriate for the group to revise their goals when they get into the problem and realize that other objectives might be productively pursued in their learning.

Setting objectives may seem awkward to the group initially, but it becomes routine when the group realizes it is essential to keeping their work efficient and productive.

The mechanics of the problem-based learning process

When a printed simulation (PBLM) or computer simulation is used by the group, there needs to be a large chalk board or equivalent (felt pen board, large paper pads) next to the small group. It is divided into four areas, the last smaller than the rest (see Figure 3). One large division entitled "hypotheses" is where the hypotheses

ideas	*facts*	*learning issues*
		future actions

Fig.3 Divisions on the chalkboard (or equivalent) prior to the problem encounter

generated by the group about the problem are listed. The next large division is entitled "patient information" where information obtained from the history, physical and laboratory tests that seems important and relevant to the hypotheses generated are listed. The last large division entitled "learning issues" is where things that need to be studied as the result of the questions, confusions, and areas of ignorance that emerge during work with the problem are listed. A last small division is entitled "future actions" where actions that the group wants to carry out in the future, usually laboratory tests, are listed as a reminder

One student is picked to be the scribe for the group. The scribe's task is to divide up the board as described and then to keep track of the group's process on the board. The scribe lists hypotheses as they are generated by members of the group, records the salient facts learned about the patient that relates to those hypotheses, and lists the learning issues identified by the group as they work with the problem. The scribe is encouraged to abbreviate copiously. It is a difficult job to be the scribe and at the same time to be an active member of the group. The task should be rotated and the others in the group should be certain that the scribe's ideas are expressed in all discussions. Until the group is used to each other and their personalities are understood, it is wise to avoid giving the scribe task to a potentially dominant member of the group, as the board and chalk can provide great power over any group discussion (the teacher reflex).

Another member of the group is given the PBLM with the task of looking up the patient's answers to history questions, findings with items of the physical examination, results of laboratory tests, and information during the patient's progress. The Users Guide for the PBLM is given to each student. It lists all the questions that anyone might want to ask any patient, all the things on physical examination anyone might want to do with any patient and all the laboratory tests that anyone might want to order. It provides the code number for finding the results to these actions in the PBLM. It takes a little time for students to get used to finding the actions they want in this guide. Initially, the tutor may take on the responsibility for finding the PBLM's code number for the actions the students wish to take on history and physical exam as they try to solve the patient's problem. However, once the students are acquainted with the PBLM, that should be a job for other members of the group, freeing the tutor to concentrate on the group's process.

The group should always be aware of the limitations of the problem simulation format they are using and work around them. Every simulation sacrifices some aspect of reality. For example, the PBLM presents the patient and the patient's problem only in words. Except for some photographs that may be included (patient's appearance, funduscopic photographs, x-rays, etc.) there are no visual, auditory, body movement, speech, or personality cues available, and students need to try and visualize the patient in their minds as much as possible. With a PBLM it is impossible to ask a series of questions as easily as is possible with a patient or standardized patient. Instead, each question or item of physical examination has to be requested one at a time. Although infuriating at times, this can be an asset for learning, as the students will have to justify each action in light of their hypotheses and not take actions just because they thought of them or are part of a menu. It disciplines their reasoning.

Presenting the problem with a standardized patient

By contrast, the standardized patient is a very faithful simulation that is in every way a patient. The use of the standardized patient allows the students to learn clinical examination and interpersonal skills in addition to reasoning skills and the acquisition of new knowledge. The "time-in/time-out" technique allows for group discussions about the problem the standardized patient presents as well as discussions about clinical and interpersonal skills.

Later, after the encounter, the standardized patient can provide students feedback on their professional manner and interpersonal skills from the patient's point of view.

When the standardized patient is used, a chalkboard is not used as is described for work with the PBLM. The chalkboard section on "patient information" represents the patient for the group. Here, the actual patient is in front of them. They should keep their own notes concerning "hypotheses" and "learning issues" and accumulated "patient facts." This puts them in the professional situation and works toward skills in note taking during the clinical encounter.

Working through the problem

Using the PBLM, the patient's presenting problem and the health care setting in which the patient is encountered are reviewed and the patient's photograph is shown around the group. The tutor, communicating at the metacognitive level, may say something such as "What could be going on with this patient?", or even more directive, "What ideas do you have about this patient's problem?", (encouraging hypothesis generation). Often students are hesitant to come up with ideas until they can ask some questions to clarify the patient's complaint. For example, a student will answer the tutor's challenge for ideas by wanting to ask the patient a question such as, "Does she have a fever?" The tutor should ask, "Why do you want to know if there is a fever?" The student will usually answer by suggesting that the patient might have an infection. The tutor can then point out to the student that he had a hypothesis in his mind-the hypothesis of a possible infection as a cause for the patient's problem and it should be put up on the board. Often the tutor has to prod the students for broader or alternative ideas by making comments such as, "Do you think the patient's problem is caused by cosmic rays or phases of the moon?"

Once there are some ideas on the board, the tutor can stimulate the students to come up with appropriate questions, and later, items on the physical examination, that will help determine which of the hypotheses generated by the group are more likely and which can be ruled out (inquiry strategy). When a student suggests a question for the patient or a physical examination item, the tutor should ask why those actions are being taken, in order to challenge the student's deductive logic in picking actions related to the hypotheses entertained.

Whenever the patient provides new information on history and physical exam, the tutor can ask what the information means and how it relates to the group's hypotheses.

After working through a number of patient problems, students may become impatient with such a team approach to asking questions, and each would like to ask a series of questions or perform the physical examination on their own to get to the heart of the problem. One technique that can help is to read the initial complaint of the patient then ask each student to write down a series of questions they would like to ask the patient and why. The students can then compare questions and the justifications for them. One student's list, or a combined list, can be chosen to get more information from the patient. When the group decides to perform the physical examination, the same technique can be used.

As the patient's responses to questions and results on items of the physical examination are obtained, the group analyzes that new information against the ideas on the board and records under "patient information" the information that is felt to be significant (analysis).

As seen in the physician's clinical reasoning process, hypotheses are being generated, an inquiry strategy developed, new data analyzed, and the significant data added to a growing synthesis of the problem on the chalkboard. The tutor stimulates the students' knowledge and thinking, guiding them through these steps in the clinical reasoning process as needed and encouraging discussion. This discussion brings out what the students already know and need to know. One advantage of a chalkboard is that all entries can be changed, eliminated, reorganized or expanded as the group progresses in their understanding of the problem.

As the group becomes more experienced in this process, the tutor progressively withdraws from the discussions and enters only when guidance may seem indicated.

Every once in a while during this process when the students seem to be getting off the track or confused about where to go next, the tutor should ask one student to summarize what has been learned about the patient problem. The student presenting the summary should not look at the chalkboard while doing this. Afterwards, the rest of the students are asked to critique the summary and add any important data that was left out. This stimulates reconsideration of the problem by all of the students. It makes sure that all students have the same problem in their minds in the same way and that no significant data have been ignored in their thinking. As time goes on and the group gets more experienced with the process, their presentation of this synthesis should become more and more concise and organized. In fact, it is valuable for them to begin summarizing the patient's case as if they were on clinical rounds using whatever protocol is required in the clinical clerkships.

A description and discussion of the synthesis gets the group back on the track. The group should be asked to review their hypotheses on the chalk board to see if any should be eliminated or changed in the light of what they have learned about the patient since the hypotheses were initially put up on the board. They should consider if new ones should be added.

Not infrequently, students express the need to do a complete history and physical on the patient in the PBLM. This could become very time consuming in the small group problem-solving process. This is a ritual that requires little cognitive effort other than memorizing a list of questions and physical examination items. This routine, menu-driven inquiry provides a small payoff, if any, in terms of understanding the patient's problem. The students' need to do this can be avoided if the tutor explains that it's assumed students will do a complete workup on patients in their clinical work. However, the challenge in problem-based learning is to develop effective prob-lem-solving skills asking those questions and performing those items of physical examination that are crucial, or have the greatest payoff in either supporting or eliminating the hypotheses being consid-ered. It helps to point out that these are the expert skills they will need as physicians in acute and emergency conditions when there is not the time or luxury of asking all questions and carrying out all examinations. Another way of handling this for the tutor is to allow the students to proceed in carrying out a complete history and physical. When they become frustrated with this seemingly endless undertaking, as they invariably do, the tutor can ask them to experiment with try-ing a more targeted approach.

As this problem-solving process is going on, the tutor should be aware of when students seem unsure of the facts they are discussing, seem confused, disagree with each other, or express that they need to understand something better as they work with the patient's problem. When any of these things occur the tutor should ask if there is a learning issue that should be listed on the chalkboard. Is there infor-mation that needs to be researched to better understand what they are discussing? Initially, it is not natural for the members of the group to be aware of learning issues as they arise in their discussions with the patient's problem. After the tutor does this prodding a few times it becomes easier for the group to recognize when they are unsure or confused and need to learn more. This conditions students to be able to recognize when they need to learn more information in their later clinical work; something that many clinicians have difficulty doing.

It is important for the tutor to make sure that the members of the group reveal the extent of the knowledge and understanding they have during their problem-solving activities and associated discussions. The students should recognize when the extent of their knowledge is insufficient and they need more information. All terms, phenomena, concepts, propositions or definitions mentioned in discussions should be defined. All explanations should be probed to the appropriate level of understanding by the tutor's liberal use of such questions as "why", "what do you mean" or "please explain." If the objective of the group is to acquire basic science information in their problem-based learning activity, this questioning should insure they carry explanations and discussions to the appropriate tissue, cellular or molecular level. These challenges by the tutor will soon be taken up by the students and they will provide similar challenges to each other in their discussions. At this time the tutor can begin to fade out of this problem-based learning process, interjecting a question now and then as appropriate.

This process continues until the group has carried the analysis of the case through history and physical as far as they can go with their own knowledge and skills. After the group has asked all the questions and performed all of the items of physical examination they feel are needed, they should discuss what laboratory test or diagnostic investigations they might want to carry out to further understand and treat the patient's problem. These can be listed on the chalkboard. It is best not to allow them to learn the results of the investigations during this first session. These results will often establish the patient's diagnosis and the students will lose interest in pursuing information about the alternative hypotheses they had about the patient problem. This will limit their motivation for learning to information related to the correct diagnosis. If they don't know the correct diagnosis and a number of the hypotheses they still have on the chalkboard at the end of the first session are felt to be possible, the range of their self-directed learning is much larger, broadening their knowledge base. This of course is consistent with clinical practice as the results of laboratory or diagnostic tests are usually not available right after being ordered.

There are two treacheries that need to be avoided in the assignment of learning issues by the students. After a while students begin to realize that increasing numbers of learning issues will translate into more work during self-directed study and will avoid acknowledging learning issues to avoid this. The other treachery is seen when students will too readily list a learning issue on the board to avoid having to think and reveal what they know or don't know in the group's discussions about a particular issue.

Commitment

This step occurs after the students have considered the most probable ideas or hypotheses they can come up with about the patient's problem. When they have asked all of the questions on history and carried out all the items of physical examination they feel are necessary or indicated and have narrowed down their ideas as to the causes for the patient's problem as far as they are able with the knowledge they have, the tutor then asks each student to make a commitment as to what he or she thinks is probably going on with the patient. When all is done, what will the patient turn out to have? Although students often feel that they do not have enough knowledge to make such a decision and would like to look up some things and order some tests, the tutor should insist that, in spite of all that, they should now make the best guess they can. What is their "gut" reaction? If they had to put down money, what would they bet on (diagnostic decision making)? This commitment provides a strong motivation for self-directed learning as the students will want to find out if their "guesses" were correct. It prepares them for the real world of practice when decisions often have to be made when data are lacking.

Reviewing learning issues

Now that the students have reasoned their way through the problem as far as possible with the knowledge and skills already possessed by the group and each have made a commitment as to what they feel is the explanation for the problem, they need to review the learning issues that have accumulated on the chalk board and decide on how they are to be tackled. The learning issues should be reviewed in the light of the objectives agreed upon in the beginning of the session. If they are in the basic science portion of the curriculum, and the identification of the basic mechanisms responsible for the patient problem as well as the normal form and function of the systems and structures involved were agreed upon objectives, the learning issues can be reviewed and focused, if necessary, to emphasize basic science learning.

The learning issues are often hastily put up on the chalkboard by the scribe during the problem-solving process with only an abbreviation or two to indicate the area of the issue. The group should see how each issue should be written to define the area and depth of study required. Now, at the end of the first session some may seem trivial or unrelated to their objectives at this point and can be eliminated. The group may also realize that there are other issues that need to be listed for study relative to the problem at hand. The group has to make a decision about breadth and depth of learning and how far beyond immediate relevance to the problem the learning should be. Those learning issues that are directly related to analyzing and understanding the problem are the most important. However, the problem may make the students realize that there are larger topics or important subject areas raised by the problem that they do not understand or fully understand, and could profitably be reviewed at this time.

Next, the group should decide on how to divide the learning issues. Although there is a tendency for students to want to research and study all the learning issues on their own, there are a number of reasons not to do this. Usually there are a large number of learning issues and if each student takes them all, the resultant learning is bound to be broad but superficial. The resources students are accustomed to using are textbooks and it will be hard to get them to use more primary sources of information when each feels there is so much to learn. Textbooks, at best, can only give an overview. It would be far more valuable for students to review original articles, online information resources, anatomical dissections, models, microscopic slides, resource faculty (assigned consultants for the curricular unit the students are in), other experts etc. as necessary in their self-directed study. The student can pursue one or two learning issues in depth using cross correlations and careful searches. The other advantage is that students with a few assigned learning issues will have the task of transferring this information effectively to the other students in the group in ways in which they will understand it and apply it to the problem at hand. This is a challenge to students' communication, team and educational skills.

Of course, the last thing students should do on return from self-directed study is to lecture each other about what they learned with particular learning issues, vitiating the whole point behind problem-based learning. One way to minimize this is to make available to the students unlimited use of xerographic copy machines so that they can bring in copies of journal articles, book pages, diagrams, and even their own study notes as follow-up resources for the other members of the group to study. Sometimes students can arrange for a resource faculty or other expert in the area of study to come into the group and comment on the way they have put the problem together and to answer questions from the group. Several students might select the same learning issue, and this encourages collaboration during self-directed study.

There are usually some learning issues that may be of such central interest to the group that they all may want to research them and then compare what they have learned. It is a general observation by most tutors that even though the students have all agreed to their own particular learning issues they also tend to do a little, perhaps superficial, reading in the area of all the others.

It is very important that students do not take on learning issues in areas in which they have prior knowledge and experience. Instead they should take on learning issues in the areas they know the least about. For example, a biology major may repeatedly take on anatomical and physiological learning issues, a biochemistry major biochemical issues, a student with a background in psychology or sociology take on learning issues in those areas, etc. It is far more important for these students to take on learning issues in areas of ignorance to extend their knowledge.

Choosing learning resources

Once the learning issues have been identified and assigned, each student should make a commitment as to the resources they intend to use in their study. Students should eventually be able to choose the most appropriate and effective resource for every particular learning need. When is a textbook, a consultant (resource faculty, faculty experts, outside experts), a computerized information search, a journal article or an online information resource the most appropriate resource? This commitment by each student sets the stage for the beginning of the second session when they return to continue with the problem and are asked to critique the resources they made a commitment to use. In this manner, skills in self-directed learning are developed and honed.

As a last step in this first session, the group then looks in their respective calendars, as does the tutor, and decides how long they should give themselves for self-directed learning. The length of time for self-directed study is determined by the extent and complexity of the learning issues chosen and the resources they plan to use. The group determines when they will meet to continue with the problem, armed with their new knowledge.

Many times tutors have asked whether it would be useful to describe to the group the steps in the clinical reasoning process used by physicians in the beginning of a problem-based learning curriculum. I prefer not to do this for two reasons. First, it is a natural problem-solving process that we all use in our life coping with the everyday ill-structured problems. We automatically generate alternative ideas or actions and seek the information we feel we need to figure out what is going on and what to do about it, and it will seem natural to the students in working with a patient problem without the need to describe it. My second reason is related to this first one, I am concerned that any prior description of a problem-solving process might sound like an artificial process that is being imposed on them. Later on, after they have become used to working with patient problems, I do describe this process and say, in essence, isn't it interesting and reassuring that we are carrying out the same reasoning process with our patient problems that expert physicians use in their clinical work?

Self-directed learning

The period of self-directed learning that follows this first session is at the heart of problem-based learning. The students are learning what they have determined is important for them to learn, and want to learn. They seek out the information on their own. They go to a variety of resource books and prior notes in their own personal collection, to faculty, to the library and to online resources with unresolved questions and a need for knowledge related to a problem they are working with and have tried to analyze on their own. They realize the information they are going after is something they do not know and should know as it relates to their being successful physicians. In contrast to assigned reading in teacher-directed learning, where maintaining the attention and interest needed to assimilate information is often a difficult labor for the student. This information that they seek on their own initiative to answer their questions literally seems to jump out of the pages or resources they are using. What the resource faculty they have consulted tells them, in answer to their questions, makes sense and is eagerly received because they want the information, and their own study has not resolved their questions. Resource faculty are often quite surprised to find the problem-based learning students more like graduate students in the quality, depth and detail of their questions. Conversations with them can be stimulating.

Medical school librarians in schools that have converted to problem-based learning describe their surprise at the remarkable increase in library use by these students, and at all hours.[53]

The students should be encouraged to collaborate in their study, working in pairs, triads or larger groups as they pool resources and discuss their understanding from the information they have acquired. In these collaborative discussions, they teach and learn from each other. Collaborative learning is enhanced by a home base for each group. In the home base, they can study and collaborate 24 hours a day. This is a room where they can bring in books, models, microscopes, computers, coffee makers etc. to support collaborative learning activities. In these home bases there should be a computer attached to the library's holdings with access to online resources.

Chapter Ten

THE AUTHENTIC PROBLEM-BASED LEARNING PROCESS (CONTINUED)

The second session with the problem following self-directed study

Resource critique

From the students' self-directed study, each is asked to describe and critique the learning resources they used. Were they the resources they intended to use? If not, why did they go to others? What were the problems with any resources used?

In their initial attempts at self-directed learning, students usually run into many difficulties. Resources can be difficult to find. Some are superficial with too little information and others too detailed with too much information. Resource faculty can be hard to track down or contact. Occasionally students can't find a satisfactory resource. The problems of each student should be discussed by the group for comment and suggestions. Every student who had problems with resources should describe them, so she or he will attack a similar learning issue differently in the future.

These discussions give the tutor an opportunity to interject challenges about the accuracy and usefulness of learning resources and information in general. They should ask students to become increasingly critical of their sources of information. The tutor should also ask how timely and up-to-date the information is that students have obtained. They should be encouraged to use primary sources of information.

Issues such as the following can be added by the tutor as the group progresses in their self-directed learning skills over the period of a unit:
- How contemporary is the information in that resource? When was the book or article published?
- What is the reliability of the information? Just because it was in the library is it a reliable resource? Who are the authors and what makes them authorities?
- When resource faculty, other experts or consultants provide information or answers, students should verify the information

they get from other resources (books, journals)?
- When should a textbook, reference book, monograph, review article, research article, or resource faculty be used as a learning resource?
- If the resource used was a research report, how appropriate was the research design and the methods used, was the data analysis appropriate, were the authors' conclusions warranted by the results obtained?
- When experts disagree (two journal articles disagree, two faculty teachers disagree, a faculty resource disagrees with a journal article or textbook, etc.), how is this to be resolved in making decisions about the patient problem?

As mentioned before, students initially will tend to use textbooks almost to the exclusion of other types of resources. It is the job of the tutor to encourage their use of other more contemporary sources of information, such as, journal articles, online resources, and resource faculty until students are comfortable with them and will use these resources when appropriate for the information sought. Developing this ability is so important for their future careers as physicians to keep up with new knowledge in their patient work. This is essential to the application of evidenced-based medicine.51 The skills needed to apply evidence-based medicine can be fostered in the discussions that occur around resource choice before self-directed learning and these discussions following self-directed learning.

Reanalysis of the patient problem in the light of the new information learned during self-directed study

Having just completed their self-directed study, the students are excited about what they have learned, the insights they now have achieved with the problem, and are eager to tell each other what they have learned. This would, in essence, create a number of mini-lectures. This would not only be boring, it would be counter productive to problem-based learning. Instead of reciting the information they have learned, students need to apply it back to the problem. This will enhance their understanding and later recall of the information learned in clinical work. This is a very important phase in the tutor's skill to make certain the students get maximum benefit from what they have learned in relation to their future career.
The students have just completed an episode of self-study to acquire

information they felt was needed to thoroughly understand and successfully analyze the patient's problem. One member of the group should summarize the facts in the patient's problem to be sure that they all agree on the data obtained about the patient prior to self-directed study. The students were more or less naive about a number of things when they first tackled the problem before self-directed learning, and those things were converted into learning issues. Now, after self-directed learning they can be considered to have expertise about the problem. The tutor can say to them in essence at this point, "Now that you are experts on this problem, let's see how you would change your hypotheses about the patient's problem.

To initiate discussion that will lead to the application, not recital, of what the students have learned, the group should review their hypotheses on the chalkboard and decide if they are still valid and whether they should be altered, extended, eliminated or new ones should be considered. Each hypothesis listed on the chalkboard should be looked at in turn for comment and discussion. As soon as a member of the group makes a suggestion about one of the hypotheses during this review—strengthening it, weakening it, changing it, or eliminating it, the tutor should inquire why he made the suggestion. This almost invariably leads to that student describing what was learned and how it applies to the patient. In the discussion that follows from this description, other members of the group are encouraged to comment, bringing their understanding of the patient's problem in the light of their new learning. From this active discussion, based on a careful review of prior hypotheses, the relevant information obtained from the self-directed study of each student can be brought to bear on those areas that caused the learning issues to be generated in the previous session. In these discussions the students can elaborate on what they learned and hand out any background materials, xerographic copies, notes, etc. that they may have prepared for later review and personal files of the others. The tutor's task is to keep this discussion going and to make sure that eventually every learning issue investigated during self-directed study by the members of the group is brought into the discussions. When the ongoing discussion offers a natural opening for a student's particular learning issue, the tutor can draw the student's information into the discussion by saying something like, "This discussion seems to be relevant to what you went off to study, what are you thoughts?"

The students may decide on the basis of new hypotheses or their discussion that other questions should have been asked of the patient and other items of physical examination performed. If so, they can then ask or perform these items to see what new information might be learned. The objective in all of this is for students to actively apply what was learned to the patient's problem, critique the accuracy of their prior knowledge and understand the adequacy of their prior problem-solving. In this manner, integrated knowledge structures are built around the contexts of patient problems in the students' minds with associations to the cues that appear in practice. Their clinical reasoning is practiced, critiqued and enmeshed with their learning. This is a most powerful part of the problem-based learning process.

When a student's presentation in these discussions becomes a lecture, it is something that the group needs to monitor and discuss. If a student has to give a formal presentation it is an opportunity to evaluate that student's ability to get peers involved in an active, interactive discussion.

Any learning issue that was researched by a student but not brought up in the patient-oriented discussion needs to be discussed before the group decides on what they have learned about the problem and where they will go with it next. It is very frustrating for a student to have studied a learning issue and then not have the opportunity to discuss it with the group.

Not infrequently the group will realize that in this application of new learning to the problem more learning issues have been created by questions as yet unanswered and by new questions raised as they attempt to understand the problem down to the cellular or molecular level. Another period of self-directed study should be negotiated, recycling through the same sequence of activities up to this point.

Summarizing what has been learned

Experienced physicians working with difficult cases can be seen to readily generate the right diagnosis and differential diagnoses to be considered. They knife in on just the right questions on history, perform the items of physical examination and order the crucial laboratory tests that sort out the differential possibilities. Yet when asked by a resident why they performed these things they are frequently unable to give any kind of a discussion of the basic or clinical science mechanisms involved, and if pushed, may just indicate that they know those actions are right. Often they will recall details of a related patient problem. Knowledge acquired in the context of active learning around a problem is stored in memory as how to or procedural knowledge. This in contrast to the knowledge acquired from readings and lectures that was memorized for later factual recall and stored as declarative knowledge that can be verbalized in response to questions. Procedural knowledge can be applied to problems but cannot be verbalized, abstracted or intellectually manipulated for adaptation to new problems. Declarative knowledge cannot be applied in work with problems, but can be verbalized in response to test questions.

Székely carried out a learning experiment that demonstrated this point.[54] He taught physics to two groups of college students using differing teaching methods. With one he used conventional didactic teaching and with the other an approach similar to problem-based learning. He deliberately chose students who had never taken a course in physics. One particular session involving the principle of angular momentum was imbedded in several days of teaching about other principles of physics, so that session was not recognized as being part of an experiment. One group learned by reading a text on the subject of angular momentum and then observed a torsion bar demonstration where they saw the dramatic increase in angular momentum that occurs when weights are shifted from the ends of the torsion bar to half way towards the point of suspension in the center. The other group, without any preparation, was asked to predict what would be observed when the wound-up torsion bar was released with the weights at the ends and then repeated with the weights shifted half way towards the point of suspension. The students were encouraged to make predictions (hypotheses) about what they would observe based on their present knowledge of physics. None were correct. The students in this group were surprised by the dramatic increase in speed (as when a spinning ice skater pulls in outstretched arms). They were asked to explain why they were not able to predict such a dramatic change in the speed of rotation. When they were unable to come up with a suitable explanation, they agreed that they should learn about the principle of physics involved. They were then given the same text on angular momentum given to the other group. Following their reading, SzÈkely discussed with them what they learned. This was done 25 years before problem-based learning was identified as an educational approach. He called it the "modern" method of learning. Few would disagree that the first group of students was taught by the traditional method and that is what he labeled that group. The second group was given the torsion bar demonstration as a problem. This teaching experiment, using the two contrasting methods was, as mentioned, imbedded in a series of physics principles that were to be learned. In this way the students would have no clue that a subsequent physics problem presented several days later to both groups was in any way related to the torsion bar principle. This time students in both groups were shown two balls of the same weight, size and color and told that one was hollow and the other one solid. When asked how that could be possible they all hypothesized that the hollow ball had to be made of denser material. Székely confirmed this with a cross-sectional drawing of each ball that indicated a dense wall in the hollow ball and the even distribution of a lesser density in the solid ball. The problem they were all given was to determine which ball was the solid one. Thirteen out of the twenty students taught in the problem-based learning mode solved the problem. Those students suggested rolling the balls down an inclined plain and the solid one would travel faster. Only four out of the twenty taught in the traditional way could solve the problem. Fortunately for us, Székely did not stop at this point with his experiment. He asked those in the problem-based learning group how they had solved the problem, what principle of physics was involved, and few could tell him. They said that the solution "just came to them." When further pressured through discussion to come up with the principle of physics involved in their solution, only a few in the problem-based learning group could relate this to what they had learned in the torsion bar demonstration. The four that solved the problem in the traditional group did recall where they had learned the principle used. He subsequently gave all students in each group a written test. One question on the test was to define angular momentum. All twenty in the traditional group could do this. None of the thirteen students that had solved the problem in the problem-based group could define angular momentum. Those in the problem-based learning group were successful in problem-solving a new problem by applying what they had learned through prior problem solving using recalled procedural knowledge, but could not recall the concepts or facts they had learned. By contrast the traditional group was quite unsuccessful in recalling and applying what they had learned to solving the problem, but were more successful in recalling the facts they had learned in a response to a written question. This is an example of "inert knowledge" described previously.

Verbalizing what has been learned

The tutor should encourage students to verbalize what they have learned through discussion so that they have the best of both methods. They are able to recall and apply the information they acquire to patient problems and also able to describe the principles and concepts behind their reasoning and treatment decisions. In this discussion they can be challenged to produce definitions, draw diagrams, make lists, model mechanisms, etc. This will help them manipulate their knowledge in work with future problems and to pass the ubiquitous written and oral questions they will always have to face in certifying examinations. This is one reason for this summary stage in the problem-based teaching sequence.

Encouraging transfer

A second phase encourages transfer of the information learned and the experience gained from one problem to a broader range of problems to which the information and experience are relevant. The students are encouraged to discuss how their new learning and experience with the present problem relate to the previous problems they have encountered in their study and how it may help them with future similar patient problems they may encounter. The writings of Spiro, Coulson, et al demonstrate the value of the "cognitive flexibility" produced in the mind of the problem solver by visiting and revisiting problems from different viewpoints.[55] Cognitive flexibility also enhances problem solving and transfer of problem solving to new and unique problems as the problem solver becomes accustomed to attacking problems from different viewpoints and adapting prior principles and facts to new settings and situations. In the process of problem-based learning the students can look at present and past problems from numerous viewpoints; anatomical, physiological, clinical, epidemiological, economical etc.

A third phase of this important stage is for the students, guided by the tutor, to develop general principles and abstractions as they see how the same or similar facts, structures, principles or processes from various disciplines apply in different settings and with different problems. They can determine how common features among different problems may suggest overarching principles. For example the problem under consideration may have shown a spastic hemiparesis with increased reflexes due to corticospinal tract lesion. Reflecting on the past problems they have seen with corticospinal tract lesions, but with different manifestations in muscle tone and weakness they could generate an overall concept of corticospinal tract function and deficit.

The students develop their own "big pictures" that faculty experts often try to provide in their lectures during traditional teaching, but to little avail as students do not have the experiences and personalized frames of reference needed to have an understanding of the significance of that big picture. Such abstractions and concepts have to be developed, as in the expert, through experience with many different instances and problems and with reflection that produce a personally constructed, and therefore owned, big picture.

Concept map

The use of a concept map is an essential final step in this stage. Using a chalkboard, the members of the group start with the patient's symptoms and signs listed at the top of the board. They then note down and connect to them the immediate factors or situations that led to each. Following this the factors that led to those factors; continuing in this manner until reaching down to the very basic mechanisms involved at the tissue, cellular or molecular levels. Doing this allows the students to see if there are missing elements in the steps going from basic causes to clinical manifestations (possibly leading to more self-directed study). This also allows them to appreciate the overall picture of the patient problem and to describe verbally the mechanism involved.

Self and peer evaluation

In this last stage of the problem-based learning process, students are asked to evaluate their own performance in four areas. These areas relate to the goals of problem-based learning. After each student has finished with a self-evaluation, the members of the group are asked to comment on the accuracy of the evaluation from their observations of the student and to make any additional evaluative comments they might have about the student's performance. These are the four areas:

Performance as a problem-solver

Since the group worked on the problem together, the challenge is for each to separate personal problem-solving activity with the problem from that of the group, reflecting what went on in their own minds, and its adequacy. Were the hypotheses generated about the problem adequate? Did the student know in his own mind what questions and examination actions should be taken with the problem (inquiry)? How well did the student put the problem together in his mind (synthesis)? Were his decisions made about the underlying processes involved and how they might be managed appropriate or correct?

Performance as a self-directed learner

Each student should address the appropriateness of the learning issues undertaken and whether appropriate resources for learning were sought and used. Was the extent and quality of the information brought back to the group satisfactory? What was the accuracy, quality and adequacy of the information? How well was it put across to the others in the reworking of the problem?

Growth in learning

Each student needs to consider how well she is progressing in her knowledge and understanding of the disciplines related to the curricular unit the group is in and the problem itself.

Performance as a member of the group

The student should evaluate his effectiveness as a member of the group. How were his interpersonal skills? How well did he support the group in its task with the problem at hand? How well did the student think he supported and contributed to the group's discussions in their ongoing work? Were other members facilitated? Were group tasks shared? Did the student feel he was too quiet or too domineering?

These are only guidelines for the possible things students might talk about in considering their own performance. Students have rarely encountered this type of activity in their previous educational or life experiences and find it initially uncomfortable and embarrassing. The tutor needs to understand these feelings, but, at the same time, encourage the students to be open and honest about their own feelings. Often the tutor has to prime them initially by asking direct questions about aspects of their performance.

After the self-assessment presented by each student, the other students in the group are then asked to comment on the student's self-assessment and to add their own comments, good or bad, about the student's performance. These comments should be supported by specific examples. The ability to provide honest, accurate and constructive feedback to a peer is even more difficult for students. In the beginning they are all very civil to each other. If, for example, during a self-assessment one student should comment on her concern that she did not get enough information to the group about the learning issue she was assigned, the others will invariably reassure her that it was a difficult topic or that there were not good resources available. The tutor should model the performance expected in providing feedback. If, indeed, this student did a poor job the tutor needs to openly comment on this with examples. More importantly, if there was a poor performance by a student that was not mentioned during self-assessment or in the subsequent comments by the other students, the tutor should comment on this poor performance. Once any group has been together for a week or so they will get beyond the usual initial civilities and become open in their criticism or support of each other. The students in the group should realize the open and honest assessment is invaluable and helps students become more effective in their goal of becoming a physician. Although not essential, self-assessment works best in a curriculum that does not have grades and uses pass/fail judgements. In this situation there is no competition between students, and they can wholeheartedly assist each other.

Whenever self-assessment or assessment by peers in the group identifies inadequacies and deficiencies, the tutor needs to ask the student how he will go about rectifying the problem identified. The other members in the group can assist in this discussion. Often students are more effective in understanding a peer's problem and can be effective in offering advice or help. Problems brought up in the group should be the group's responsibility. It is inappropriate for the tutor to counsel a student in the group outside of the group.

Self-assessment requires students to monitor their own performance and to judge its adequacy. The development of this ability is central to effective life-long, self-directed learning skills. Practicing physicians need to be aware of inadequacies in their daily work to be able to recognize the need for more learning. They should be willing and able to update knowledge and skills to keep contemporary in practice and meet new challenges that will always evolve in practice. In addition, the ability to provide constructive feedback to others is essential for working effectively in health care or research teams.

As will be seen later, self and peer assessment is a principal source of student assessment in problem-based learning.

Tutors should also assess their own performance as the group's tutor with feedback from the group.

Moving towards individual, as opposed to group learning

In the above sequences, the students work as a group to take advantage of peer support and the wealth of accumulated knowledge that occurs in collaborative learning. They learn to work effectively in team settings. However, once the students have become proficient in this learning process and have developed an experience with a sufficient number of patient problems, they can and should begin to work individually with patient problems as they move towards individual work on clinical services. They use the same sequence of activities in their individual problem work. Later they can confer, compare and discuss their individual approaches to the same problem, entering as a group just before the step where the group summarizes what has been learned.

Parallel clinical activity

The sequence of activities in problem-based learning using problem simulations such as PBLMs and standardized patients is reinforced from the first week of medical school by at least a half day of clinical experiences every week. In these experiences, the students should be actively involved in working with real patients, learning to interview and examine them and presenting their findings and thoughts for discussion with physicians. As much as is possible, the patients they work with should present problems that correlate with their curricular unit. This activity allows them to transfer what is learned in their problem-based learning sessions from patient simulations to the real world of clinical work and further extends their learning. It would be valuable for the students to meet with the same clinical preceptor each week for these experiences as she can help them develop their clinical skills in a progressive manner.

Relating the process to the objectives for problem-based learning

Now that the sequence of activities that occurs in problem-based learning has been described; we can review the educational objectives that were to be addressed simultaneously by this problem-based learning process. These are somewhat modified from those described in Chapter VII.

1) The acquisition of an extensive knowledge base that is:

a) Integrated from multiple discipline/subject areas
b) Retained in long term memory
c) Structured for application to patient problems
d) Recalled in association with patient problem cues that occur in clinical contexts
e) Enmeshed with the clinical reasoning process used in clinical practice

This objective is addressed by the use of a patient problem as the basis for learning, the identification of learning issues leading to active learning in multiple disciplines, the application of new knowledge from these disciplines to an understanding of the problem, and the summarization and integration of what has been learned relative to that problem as well as other patient problems presented in the curriculum and experienced in correlated clinical experiences.

2) The development of clinical reasoning skills

This objective is addressed through:
a) The design of patient simulations that permit the application of the clinical reasoning or problem-solving process in the attempt to understand and manage the patient problem,
b) The guidance provided by the tutor in this process, and
c) The critique of the students' reasoning with a particular patient problem following self-directed study.

3) The development of independent, self-directed learning skills

This objective is addressed through the identification of learning issues and the learning resources needed, self-directed study, the critique of resources used, the application of learning to the analysis of the patient problem, and self-evaluation.

4) The development of skills in history taking, physical examination, patient education, communication and interpersonal skills

In their work with the standardized patient, the student's interpersonal skills are practiced and critiqued by both peers and the standardized patient. Interpersonal skills are also stressed in their parallel clinical work.

5) The development of a continual drive to learn, question and understand

This is addressed by:
a) The obvious relevance of what has to be learned for the practice of medicine,
b) The relevance of what has been taken on as learning issues to the learning needs of the individual student,
c) The commitment made by each student about the nature of the patient problem before self-directed study,
d) The fact that the students are working with real medical problems as they learn, and
e) The motivation and curiosity provoked by medical problems in general.

6) An early immersion into the culture and values of medicine as a profession to become aware of such things as:

a) The ambiguities of practice and the limits of knowledge
b) Experts can hold differing opinions
c) The responsibilities and obligations of the physician in caring for individual patients and communities of patients
d) The moral and ethical dilemmas of medicine
e) The complexities of health care delivery and the financial burdens and inequities involved

This is addressed by learning in the context of patient problems, using the terminology and thinking processes required in clinical work. The students go to multiple sources of information, often conflicting, and have to resolve the conflict for themselves. They have to make decisions about the patient and the management of the problem in the face of inadequate and conflicting information. They learn that there are many times no answers for their questions about the patient and the basic science issues involved. As all learning stems from patient problems, the moral and ethical dilemmas become learning issues in themselves and part of the active learning process.

7) The development of team skills

This is accomplished in the group process where common problem-solving, active discussion, collaborative learning, self-evaluation and peer evaluation are exercised.

Chapter Eleven

THE AUTHENTICITY OF PROBLEM-BASED LEARNING

An authentic educational program is one that requires students to carry out the same activities while learning that are used and valued in the real world outside of school. Problem-based learning is an authentic educational method from several different viewpoints.

1) The patient problem simulations used in problem-based learning present the students with the problem-solving and learning challenges of clinical practice.

2) The problems are always based on actual patients.

3) More importantly, the sequence of activities in the problem-based learning process, described previously, undertaken by the group

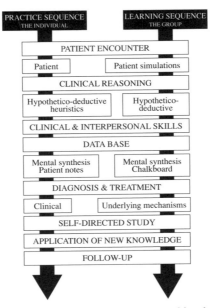

Fig.4 Comparing the sequence of activities in problem-based learning and clinical practice

as they work with the simulated problem, is authentic in that it is the same sequence of activities or behaviors that physicians undertake with a patient (see Figure 4).

For example:

A physician encounters the patient as an unknown with initially insufficient information to come to a conclusion about providing care without an investigation of the patient's problem through history, physical and laboratory tests. Physicians have to do this with the knowledge and skills they possess at the time.

> In problem-based learning the small group encounters the patient simulation as an unknown with insufficient information to come to any satisfactory conclusion about providing care without carrying out an investigation through history and physical. The students in the group have to do this with the knowledge and skills they possess at the time, as there was no prior preparation or advance knowledge about the patient's problem provided to them.

In their work with the patient, physicians employ the hypothetico-deductive reasoning process if the patient's problem is unfamiliar, unusual, or confusing. Physicians may employ short cuts (or heuristics) with a problem, with which they have had many prior experiences, using a few hypotheses and a limited number of actions to come to a diagnostic and treatment conclusion.

> In their work with the patient problem, the students in the group practice and develop their hypothetico-deductive process. As students, they are neophytes with little to no prior experience with a similar patient problem and need to perfect their use of the hypothetico-deductive reasoning process. Heuristics may emerge in the group's problem solving later on in the curriculum. In this activity the tutor guides the students through all the stages of the hypothetico-deductive process.

Physicians use clinical and interpersonal skills to obtain the information needed while reasoning through the patient problem and to establish an effective professional working relationship with the patient.

> Using the standardized patient, (augmented by parallel clinical activity) the students learn, practice and develop their clinical and interpersonal skills. The standardized patient can provide students with direct feedback about communication, interpersonal and educational skills.

During the patient workup, physicians keep developing a synthesis of the important facts about the patient in their heads along with the diagnostic and treatment ideas being entertained as the workup progresses. This synthesis is often augmented by notes on a patient chart. This mental synthesis is used at the end of the workup to record the case (database, diagnostic ideas and a treatment plan for the patient).

> The group keeps a record of their hypotheses and important data obtained from the patient simulation on a chalkboard. During their work with the problem, a student is often challenged to describe the patient synthesis in her or his head, and the others are asked to comment on the synthesis from their own perspective. With the standardized patient (and the patients they encounter clinically) they keep these facts as a growing synthesis in their heads.

Physicians conclude their encounter with the patient and come to a decision about the probable working diagnosis(es) and an appropriate management.

> When the group has carried their workup of the patient's problem as far as they are able, they should make a commitment as to the underlying mechanisms or pathophysiology involved in the patient's problem. They can also describe what laboratory or diagnostic tests they want to order to continue with their investigation, and treat the patient.

During the workup, physicians often recognize that there are things that they do not know and need to review relative to diagnosing or managing the problem the patient presents. As a result, journals, books, computerized information resources, colleagues, and consultants are used through self-study to acquire the information needed.

> During their work with the patient the students, initially guided by the tutor, identify areas of ignorance or confusion and list on the board the areas of information they need to acquire (learning issues). When their work is concluded with the patient's problem, they each decide on learning issues they will address in their own self-study and the resources they will use.

In a follow-up encounter with the patient, physicians apply what has been learned through self-study to the ongoing care of the patient.

> When the students return from their self-directed study, they apply what they have learned to a reanalysis of the patient's problem. In this process, the students criticize their prior knowledge and thinking, reflect on what they have learned and its application to future practice and they evaluate themselves (it would be highly desirable if all practicing physicians would do this-certainly some do).

The term authentic learning is most appropriate for problem-based learning as the problems are authentic and the learning sequence requires the very skills and knowledge that will need to be developed and employed in medical practice. Learning that is not authentic requires the student to use activities in learning that involve skills and knowledge not needed or useful in the real world. Rote memorization of vast amounts of information in an isolated discipline to perform well on written examinations, or listening passively to a series of lectures are examples of education that is not authentic.

Chapter Twelve

TWO COMMON CONCERNS OF MEDICAL TEACHERS

"Where is the curriculum in problem-based learning?"

This is perhaps one of most often asked questions about problem-based learning. Medical teachers considering the possible change to problem-based learning are concerned about the seeming lack of a defined curriculum. The students are seen to decide on their own what they want to learn and there is no assurance that they will learn all that is important in their all-too-brief time in medical school. The faculty in a problem-based learning curriculum are seen to be ignoring their responsibility for determining what students should learn.

This is the usual discomfort of teachers used to teacher-centered learning. Despite the fact that students in problem-based learning are given progressively increasing responsibility for their own learning so that they will be able to continue learning on their own after graduation, there is an established curriculum. The important blend of individual responsibility for learning and the existence of a defined curriculum are achieved by providing the students with appropriate and carefully chosen problems that will stimulate them to learn what is important and relevant. Problem-based learning provides the students with the skills they need to make appropriate learning decisions on their own. In this way they can adapt their learning to meet their own interests and particular learning needs. This is accomplished through the following linchpins.

Selection of problems

The patient problems and community health problems used in any section of the curriculum are carefully chosen to inevitably lead the student into the areas of learning desired by the faculty. They are chosen to raise the learning issues considered important by the faculty responsible for that portion of the curriculum. In addition, the problems chosen represent those the students will encounter in future practice ensuring that what is learned is relevant and contemporary to the practice of medicine. The process of choosing problems for problem-based learning is considered in more detail in Chapter XVIII.

Preparation and orientation of the tutor

The tutors chosen for a particular unit or section of the curriculum are informed by the unit designers about each problem used in the unit. They are told why the problem was chosen, the expected learning issues that the students will generate, and points about particular features of the problem or special learning resources that might be available. This is provided as a printed resource. With this information, the tutor can guide the students with questions and challenges at a metacognitive level (see *The Tutorial Process*[1]) so that the students will raise the learning issues appropriate for the problem. This does not prevent the students from going far beyond the expectations of the faculty or from entering valuable areas of learning that may not even have been anticipated by the faculty. The skillful tutor can provide this subtle but important guidance without student awareness and without diminishing their responsibility for learning.

Review by discipline consultants

Consultants from the various disciplines involved review the curriculum periodically to ensure that the problems used will cover the important concepts from their particular subject or discipline and to keep up with changes in their respective fields.

Guides given to the students

To give the students the information they need to assume more responsibility for their own learning, they are provided with a number of guides to help them make their own decisions about what should be learned in their work with a particular problem, and to what depth.

In the back of each PBLM, the faculty from the various disciplines involved in the problem provides the learning issues they feel the students should take on in their problem-related, self-directed study. The students refer to these only after their work with the problem has been finished and they have dealt with all the learning issues they felt appropriate in their self-directed study. When they review these learning issues listed by the faculty, it is important for the tutor to emphasize that they are listed there, not as a prescription, but as a suggestion. It indicates the faculty's opinion and is there for the student's information and possible value. The usual experience is that students find that they have already raised most of the learning issues suggested. They may discover some that they did not think of and feel are important. In this case, they can continue with the problem and address these issues or take them up with the next problem.

Every student is provided with the educational objectives, stated in behavioral terms, for each curricular unit. The objectives do not indicate the content that is to be learned but, instead, describe how the problems in the unit are to be approached and the depth and areas of learning expected. There is an example of curricular objectives for a unit in Appendix I.

The content outline for the United States Medical Licensing Examination (USMLE) Step I is provided to the student. This examination has to be passed to obtain licensure in the United States and is characteristically taken at the completion of the second and last preclinical year. Students in a problem-based curriculum are usually concerned about the adequacy of their readiness for this multiple-choice examination since their learning in problem-based learning is designed to prepare them for their career as a physician and not to regurgitate all the information on a multiple choice examination that an external examining agency might feel they ought to know. As pointed out by Vernon and Blake, traditional programs seem to have an advantage with respect to this examination.[10] Teaching that stresses the memorization of information prepares students for tests that ask them to regurgitate or display (as opposed to use) the information. To help alleviate this concern and to combine the problem of board preparation with their self-directed learning, they have this content outline to refer to in their self-directed learning. In this way they can extend or modify what they are studying to cover the expectations of the examination.

All these linchpins ensure that there is a curriculum and that the basic philosophy of problem-based learning is not violated in the process of ensuring that the curriculum is intact.

"Problem-based learning is not an efficient way to learn"

Another commonly voiced concern by faculty considering a change to problem-based learning is that it does not seem efficient. They are concerned that the students spend too much time playing around with a patient problem, coming up with incorrect hypotheses, and not having the basic science knowledge that is needed. They wander around with a variety of learning issues that do not seem pertinent to what they should be learning, etc. They think it would be far more efficient just to give the students what they need to know instead of having them waste all that time in those small group process activities.

Whenever efficiency is mentioned as a concern by faculty in this context it usually refers solely to efficiency in the acquisition of information. The question tacitly assumes that this is the only objective for student learning. The acquisition of information is only one of many objectives in problem-based learning, all of which are being addressed in this learning process. Looked at in the context of all of these objectives for problem-based learning; acquiring effective reasoning, self-directed learning and team skills and how to apply what is learned to the care of patients, the sequence of activities in the small group can be seen as efficient. In addition, faculty who raise this issue are either unaware or forget that over 80% of what is told students in a lecture, in contrast to information students dig out for themselves, will be forgotten or not accessed in later practice. Much that is recalled can't be applied. Telling students what they need to know is really not efficient at all, but very inefficient.

Chapter Thirteen

INTEGRATING OTHER LEARNING METHODS INTO PROBLEM-BASED LEARNING

The small group tutorial should not be thought of as the exclusive method of teaching in problem-based learning. It is the centerpiece as it brings to light the skills and knowledge of all students, permits interactions between students and the faculty tutor that are unmatched in other formats, and permits active, collaborative, problem oriented learning. However, other learning methods have other educational advantages and should be incorporated into problem-based learning in ways that will capture their unique advantages without competing with or diluting the effectiveness of problem-based learning. For example, there are a number of reasons for using the occasional lecture.

- There may be a visiting expert who has information you would like to have the students hear and is around for too short a period of time for the students to interact in any other way.

- There is information that you want the students to know about that may not yet be relevant to any patient problem and yet represents an area of recent research development that you feel will be important for them to be aware of as it may become medically relevant.

- There is someone on the faculty who can put over a difficult concept, relative to what the students are now studying, in a way that cannot be obtained from the available literature. Watch out for this one as it could grow to a lecture series. If this lecturer presents new, valuable or unavailable information, you should ask that person to provide or make a learning resource for the students in the future that conveys the concept. Students can use the resource in their self-directed study.

- There is someone on the faculty who has charisma and is obviously so in love with his or her field that it would be inspiring for the students to hear.

Not infrequently, students in a problem-based curriculum will request a lecture in an area of common concern related to their problem work. In this instance the lecture's value is enhanced by being a student-centered learning experience as the information in the lecture is provided at the time they feel it is needed in their ongoing work.

Laboratory experiences should be integrated into a problem-based learning curriculum. These experiences can give the student an appreciation of the thinking that goes into research, the technical problems involved, and the awareness that facts are no more than the best hypothesis at the moment. Any laboratory experience should be related to the unit the students are in and reinforce their problem-related learning. Ideally, laboratory experiences should be available to all student groups as an option in their learning. The anatomy laboratory at McMaster provided the students with a range of prosected cadavers, mounted cross sections, slides and specimens all related to the unit in which students were working. The students were permitted to perform dissections as they wished with faculty guidance as desired. At Southern Illinois University the students also have access to prosected cadavers and a similar range of anatomical materials related to the unit of study they are in. A full time member of the anatomy faculty is available to these students to assist in cadaver review, their own dissections and histology study.

The same integrative approach applies to learning technical procedures such as venipuncture and seminars on topics central to their ongoing learning.

The secret to integrating other educational methods such as lectures into the curriculum is to ask all small groups to avoid certain hours every day, such as, for example 10 to 12 noon when scheduling their group meetings. This allows the unit coordinator to insert these other learning experiences, even at the last minute.

Chapter Fourteen

VARIABLES THAT CAN ALTER THE EFFECTIVENESS OF PROBLEM-BASED LEARNING

In designing a problem-based learning curriculum it is often tempting to take short cuts or to negotiate compromises. Financial constraints, time constraints, faculty resistance to change, and inadequate support by other teachers often present difficult barriers. Many of the areas where short cuts or compromises can easily occur are listed here. You need to be aware of the effect of these variations from authentic problem-based learning. Kelson and Distlehorst sent a questionnaire to all schools in the US that claimed to be using problem-based learning. Their study shows the reliability that is present in a number of the variables listed here.[14]

Problem design

The development of the clinical reasoning process is a major goal in problem-based learning. This requires that the problems used present to the students in the same way they do clinically with only the information that is initially available. It also requires that the problem format allow for free inquiry by the students. Well structured problems, such as case reports or write-ups and case vignettes, although easier to create, will not challenge the students' clinical reasoning process fully and allow them to practice it. Standardized (simulated) patients and PBLMs meet this requirement.

Facilitatory skills of the tutor

Every school with a problem-based learning curriculum recognizes that the skill of the tutor is central to the success of the method. These skills are fully described in the companion text to this book *The Tutorial Process*.[1] Adequate training for this role is crucial to problem-based learning success. It is not enough for teachers to understand the role; they should be able to practice it.

Grades versus pass/fail

Letter or number grades rank students and therefore tend to promote competition among students. In some medical schools using grades, students have been known to deliberately mislead other students in order to get the better grade. This competition is antithetical to what is wanted in problem-based learning and inhibits students learning from each other and helping each other. The students are expected to work collaboratively on learning issues and the understanding of the problem. They should assist and instruct each other as they learn. This prepares them for the real world of practice where they will always be working in teams and expected to work together effectively around patient problems and to learn from and teach colleagues and other health professionals. It seems doubtful that any truly successful problem-based learning curriculum can be carried out if grades are required.

The amount of information students are given didactically before problem-based learning begins

Many teachers are uncomfortable starting directly with problem-based learning. They feel that the students should have some knowledge before they can be expected to undertake solving a problem. As has been pointed out by Des Marchais, some of this feeling may be due to a misunderstanding of the students' task relative to the problems presented.[7] Students are not expected to be able to solve the problems. Instead, the problems are used as a stimulus for learning. The students are being asked to analyze them to see if they understand the normal and pathophysiologic mechanisms or psychobiological dynamics involved. If they can't, they are asked to go to the relevant basic sciences resources to obtain the information they need. Other faculty feel that the students' work in their unit would be far more efficient if they were given background information, an overview of the disciplines involved in the unit, the terminology they need to understand, and some concepts basic to understanding the problems in the unit. This is, in essence, a scaffolding on which their subsequent problem-based learning could be based. There is nothing wrong with this point of view if the initial orientation is truly limited to an overview, important terminology, and important references. But it shouldn't be necessary.

There are potentially two problems associated with allowing an initial period of learning before undertaking problem-based learning. If faculty are permitted to give introductory information about the unit for, say, two days, they will invariably discover they want to have more introductory time in the next iteration of the unit. It will be difficult to hold the line and prevent the unit from slowly becoming more conventional-a position of comfort for faculty uncomfortable and unsure about problem-based learning. Gradually, more and more information that should be learned in a problem-based manner is presented in lecture format. The second problem refers back to the objectives for problem-based learning. If it is felt important for student learning to be organized around patient problems and enmeshed with the clinical reasoning process to better ensure recall and application in clinical work, then why should some information be learned with didactic, passive learning? In those curricula where the students start the very first day with problem-based learning, they do well. Terminology is learned as it arises in their work and is better remembered and used. Overviews of the subject developed by the students themselves, in small group discussions after working with a few problems in the unit are far better appreciated and integrated with their learning.

Competition with traditional courses

Many problem-based learning curricula were initially designed to be alternative or parallel curricula with an aliquot of students separated from the standard curriculum. Fewer have been designed as a total curriculum conversion to problem-based learning. Both forms may involve the preclinical years only or the entire curriculum. However, before undertaking either, many faculty wish to develop a pilot problem-based learning curriculum to see how well it works, to judge whether they want to make a greater commitment, and to let skeptical faculty evaluate it in action. Whenever a problem-based curriculum is designed to run concurrently with a standard curriculum or is added on to a standard curriculum, the quality of the problem-based learning experience is severely compromised, and both faculty and students alike become discouraged, confused and overwhelmed. They are not able, in this circumstance, to have any appreciation of what a problem-based curriculum really has to offer and may conclude that it is undesirable. The reasons for this are obvious, yet faculty will try to do this to avoid having to make serious alterations in their present curriculum.

If the students are in a standard curriculum they always have too much to learn in the time available, and little time will be set aside for self-directed study in the problem-based curriculum. The next scheduled examination, report, or presentation in the standard curriculum will take precedence over what, by contrast, seems optional time in the problem-based section of the curriculum. If the problem-based exercise is an addition to their ongoing work, the negative reactions are even worse, as the conventional curriculum is already too demanding. Added to this is the fact that both teachers and students alike are confused as to what is expected. At one time the students are expected to memorize and regurgitate what the teacher has given them and at another to tackle a problem, determine on their own what they should learn, and dig it out for themselves. The role of the teacher is equally confusing as to when they should give information and when they should facilitate learning. Almost all successful problem-based learning undertakings have been designed so that the block of time devoted to problem-based learning is free of any other curricular demands on the students. The degree to which there is competition diminishes the potential effectiveness of the problem-based learning experience.

The length of the problem-based learning experience in a pilot program

Although most functioning problem-based learning curricula run for more than two years, the length of any pilot or experimental problem-based learning experience also has an effect on the results that might be expected. Problem-based learning is a totally new and often unfamiliar approach to teaching/learning and represents a tremendous change for both students and teachers. It takes a while to get used to the demands and the advantages of the system. The students have to learn to reason, analyze, develop learning issues, dig out information on their own, and get used to not having the teacher tell them what is to be learned and whether they are right or wrong in their thinking. They also have to assess themselves. All this is threatening and uncomfortable. The teacher has to stop giving students information, despite all urges to do this, and, instead, facilitate their learning. The teacher is unsure as to whether they will learn the right things. It takes many weeks for teachers and students alike to get comfortable and begin to see the real excitement and advantages to problem-based learning. Also, as pointed out in The Tutorial Process, newly formed small groups in problem-based learning are initially very civil and well-mannered, but after three to four weeks, interpersonal problems invariably develop among students and teacher and they will have to be worked out for the group to run smoothly. All this means that any problem-based learning experience that runs for only a few weeks is a set up for frustration and failure. Any pilot problem-based learning experience should be at least six or more weeks in length. There is no reason why any discipline cannot be taught by problem-based learning.

Disciplines taught outside of problem-based learning

In a number of problem-based learning curricula there are disciplines that are taught in a traditional manner outside problem-based learning. In some schools this is anatomy, in others it is biochemistry or some other discipline. This is usually because the faculty of that discipline will not accept problem-based learning as an appropriate way for their discipline to be taught, or they are unable to see how their subject can be integrated with learning around patient problems. One of the values of problem-based learning is its ability to cause information from different disciplines to be integrated in the mind of the learner and structured around patient problems so that information will be recalled and applied in clinical practice. A subject that remains outside of problem-based learning weakens this advantage of problem-based learning.

The degree to which students are responsible for their own learning

An essential element of problem-based learning is the development of effective and efficient self-directed learning skills to enable students to educate themselves the rest of their professional careers, to meet new problems, and to keep contemporary in their knowledge. This objective requires students to be treated as adults and results in one of the most exciting collegial aspects of problem-based learning for both students and teachers. Despite this recognition, many problem-based learning curricula do not truly honor this objective and in many subtle ways are still teacher-centered, making the student, to some degree, still directly dependant on the teacher for learning. In some, the students are given the learning issues for the problems they encounter. In others, during scheduled resource sessions, resource faculty teach the students what they feel the students should know about the problem they are studying. The poorly trained or poorly oriented tutor may become directive in the small group and end up directly teaching by either giving the students information she or he feels the students should know, correcting them when they are wrong in their thinking, or asking pointed questions to show them that they are lacking in a specific area of knowledge. All problem-based learning curricula need to closely monitor the many ways in which the teacher-centered, parental approach to teaching works its way back into the process, as it is an all-too-easy reflex behavior for faculty.

The degree to which the small group meetings are on fixed schedules

It is hard for faculty to get rid of their conventional teaching reflexes, and scheduling student activity is one of these time-honored, unquestioned activities. This is important when teachers' contributions for lectures, presentations, rounds, or seminars have to be coordinated for a large class of students. It has no value in small group learning where the students and the tutor can schedule their own meetings. This flexibility is important as the time it takes to get to the bottom of a particular problem in a group meeting can vary tremendously depending on the knowledge the group brings to the problem. After working through a few problems in a unit, the students may acquire enough of an understanding to go through subsequent problems in a shorter period of time. A new problem in a new unit may require a number of hours and perhaps several group meetings; a later problem may only require an hour. The number and complexity of the learning issues that may be generated vary in a similar manner, and some of the resources that were chosen in self-directed learning may require more time. Small group learning cannot be handled in a Procrustean manner as it may weaken the depth of learning and inhibit the students from exploring interesting areas of learning that were stimulated by the problem. Scheduling also inhibits the use of busy research or clinical faculty from participating as tutors. If the small group can schedule their own times for meeting, they can adapt to the tutor's schedule. This also allows students flexibility for scheduling clinical work during the unit.

Only initial orientation meetings, recurrent meetings of all problem-based learning students and tutors to review any problems or issues, and examinations need to be scheduled. As mentioned previously, if you would like to integrate certain lectures, laboratory experiences or seminars into the problem-based learning curriculum, the groups can be asked to avoid certain hours on certain days in their ongoing scheduling.

Assessment methods used

Students will study in ways appropriate to pass any examination given to them, regardless of the way learning experiences may be structured, problem-based or otherwise. Teachers will always teach in ways that will facilitate students passing the examinations, regardless of how the teaching methods are designed. This is especially true for any examinations that contribute to the students' grade or ability to pass (summative examinations). Unfortunately, this is also true of examinations that may only be given to provide feedback to students about their progress, when students are told that the exam will not contribute to their grade or ability to pass (formative examinations). Students are always unsure about any examinations provided by their teachers. Therefore, if the examinations given in a problem-based learning curriculum or unit ask for the memorization and regurgitation of facts that the faculty feel students should know, the students will try and determine what it is that the teachers will expect them to know. As a result they will begin to memorize facts for their own sake. This seriously diminishes their attention to problem-based learning and self-directed learning around the problem. Assessment should reinforce the objectives of a problem-based learning curriculum and assess problem solving, the application of facts to a patient problem, and self-directed learning. The next chapter deals with this in more detail, as assessment is a very important variable in the effectiveness of problem-based learning.

Chapter Fifteen

ASSESSMENT IN PROBLEM-BASED LEARNING

Assessment drives any curriculum. There is no one other component in an educational program that has such a powerful effect on the way students study and the way teachers teach. Students have learned since their early grades that passing the tests in a course is the requirement for promotion. Their study methods are aimed at passing the tests. Part of the success in passing tests is knowing what the teacher wants or will expect. Teachers will teach students in ways that best ensures they pass the tests. If recalling or recognizing facts is required, they will give students facts to memorize.

Even though you emphasize to students that you expect them to learn through problem work and self-directed study in your problem-based learning course, it won't happen if you test the students with multiple choice questions or essay questions that assess what you feel students should have learned. Instead, they will try and guess what you will put on the test, what you think is important for them to learn, and they will go about memorizing that information in ways that will help them recall it on your test.

Since assessment has the whip hand it is essential that your tests and all assessment measures designed for your problem-based learning curriculum will influence the student to learn in ways consistent with the problem-based learning method. This means that you should not assess the recall and recognition of facts for their own sake, but, instead, the recall and application of facts in the context of work with a patient problem. It also means that you need to assess their evolving problem solving skills and self-directed learning skills.

Another and difficult challenge in the design of assessment in problem-based learning is that the assessment should be student-centered and not teacher centered. You can't expect the students to become responsible for their own learning in the curriculum and then provide a test in which the teacher has determined what the students should have learned. The development of self-directed learning skills will be undermined, as the students will study what they think the teacher wants them to know in preparation for the test. Tests in problem-based learning should not require any preparation on the part of the students.

Assessment in the small group

As described in the chapters on the problem-based learning process, an invaluable assessment procedure based on rich data is carried out within the small group in the final, self and peer assessment stage. At the completion of each problem every student has to evaluate his own problem-solving skills, self-directed learning skills, team skills and growth in knowledge followed by a critique from peers and the tutor. This is an informal exercise at the end of every problem encounter and is a formal discussion with a written assessment at the end of every unit. It is an assessment that is consistent with problem-based learning's objectives and fully supports the method.

The information brought back to the group by each student, and the references used, can indicate the quality of each student's self-directed learning skills. The collaborative work that goes on among students during self-directed learning time allows students the opportunity to observe the quality of each other's work and thinking. The internal motivation and drive of each student is quite apparent over time, as is acculturation of each to the professional values of medicine. In the group's intensive ongoing learning activities, day after day, each student's capabilities are clearly exposed. This rich information can be maximized by the tutor's deliberate attention to all aspects of each student's performance.

The areas assessed represent the educational goals of problem-based learning (problem solving, self-directed study, and team skills). As an attitude of open and honest assessment is established during ongoing work it becomes an effective and powerful assessment tool. This constant self and peer assessment exercise develops the valuable skills of self-assessment and the ability to critique peers in each student.

As rich and powerful as this intragroup assessment is, however, there are blind spots. The tutor and the other students in the group never observe members of the group employ clinical, interpersonal and patient-educational skills. Except for the group's use of standardized patients, the individual student's development of these evolving clinical skills with patients cannot be assessed.

If a tutor is not observant or skilled, the inadequacies of an individual student may not be noticed, as others in the group may inadvertently compensate for that student's inadequacies in their eagerness to make their own comments when that student hesitates or is unclear. The other students' observations may not be harvested at the end of each problem if a tutor has not developed a spirit of openness within the group. Despite the power of this self and peer assessment activity, even when well done, it is sometimes very difficult to accurately assess the extent of an individual student's knowledge base and her ability to apply their knowledge to patient problems.

Therefore, an objective assessment of each student's knowledge base, self-study skills and reasoning abilities at the end of every curricular unit, using an external examination of each student independent of the group provides a complementary assessment and a cross check to the tutorial group's assessment. If the external assessment is consistent with the tutorial assessment, both faculty and students are reassured. If there is a discrepancy between the group's report on a student and the student's performance on a formal, external test, further analysis needs to be made of that student's ability.

Formal, external assessment of student performance in problem-based learning

In designing an external, objective assessment method to augment and complement tutorial group assessment, the first question is what skills, capabilities or competencies should be assessed? The next question is what tools are available to assess those capabilities? And finally, how should assessment be packaged or designed?

Things to be assessed in problem-based learning

The extent of the students' knowledge base, especially in the basic sciences, and their ability to recall and apply that knowledge in work with a patient's problem is preeminent. The effectiveness and efficiency of their problem solving or clinical reasoning skills and their self-directed learning skills are an integral part of that ability and needs to be assessed. Capabilities that can't be assessed in the tutorial group and are an important part of the students' preparation to be effective physicians; such as, clinical skills, interpersonal and patient education skills need to be assessed. Testing these capabilities in the context of patient problems supports the educational process of problem-based learning.

Tools for assessment in problem-based learning

This list of tools for student assessment in problem-based learning is not intended to be all-inclusive. It serves as an orientation to the range and possibilities for tools that can be used to design assessment procedures. There is an extensive literature associated with most of these tools where their use and psychometrics are covered in greater depth.

Multiple choice questions (MCQs)

In problem-based learning, it would be inappropriate to use MCQs to test student recall of facts or concepts for their own sake. An encyclopedic knowledge base is of no use in and of itself and is no assurance that the knowledge can be recalled or used in the context and activities of care of patients.

If MCQs are incorporated during problem solving interactions with a patient problem in a simulation format such as a standardized patient, computer or PBLM they can assess the knowledge students recall and apply in the activities and contexts of patient care. Questions can ask the diagnoses being considered, interpretation of data from the patient or laboratory tests, management plans considered. The advantages of MCQs lie in easy scoring, their seeming objectivity, their reliability and the breadth of knowledge they can assess. Still the problems of cueing remains with the use of MCQs as students may be offered alternatives they might have never recalled or entertained. This drawback can be minimized using long lists of multiple options for the student to consider with some close to being right, some wrong and some very wrong along with the right ones.

Modified essay questions (MEQs)

The modified essay question uses a short fill in answer such as: "The diagnoses you are considering in your patient are _____." They avoid the problem of cueing the students by having the correct alternative available, as in MCQs, truly testing recall of information instead of recognition. They are, again, reasonably easy to score and reliable.

Essay questions

These are excellent ways to probe a student's knowledge, reasoning, organization, and ability to express and communicate. They become difficult for testing a number of students as they take a heavy toll on teacher time and issues of scoring and reliability become a concern, especially if there is more than one person scoring students answers.

Oral questions

This is an unquestionably effective tool for assessing the knowledge base, thinking and ability to communicate of the individual student. If it is to be used on a group of students or a class, the examiners have to have a carefully designed protocol to follow to ensure consistency and be trained to carry it out. Scoring involves far less objectivity and more judgement. Reliability is a concern.

Sequential management problems

Sequential management problems are written patient problems that present an initial packet of information about the patients and then ask the student questions about what has been revealed using any of the above forms (MCQs, MEQs, essay and oral questions). Questions can be asked about hypotheses considered, questions that should be asked of the patient, interpretation of symptoms described etc. Then the student is given another packet with further information about the patient, and the process goes on. This tool can assess knowledge applied to the problem and some aspects of problem solving, although very limited as the student cannot inquire and get back information from the patient. The students' problem solving strategies cannot be fully evaluated.

Modified PBLMs

The PBLM (see Appendix II) can be modified for testing a group or class of students. Students can be given a way to record their inquiries and their responses to the information they get from the patient. In the process they can be asked to indicate their hypotheses, learning issues, etc. With available computer technology (such as the DxR described below) the patient presentation, recording of student inquiry strategy and thinking is easier to accomplish.

DxR[43]

The DxR is a computerized patient simulation based on the PBLM but designed to assess student problem solving and is becoming available on compact disks and on the World Wide Web. It presents visuals; such as, x-rays, scans, and the patient's appearances. The interview and examination of the patient is enhanced by graphics (such as putting the stethoscope on the patient's chest and hearing the cardiac sounds). It queries the students' thinking at all stages of their problem solving approach. All of the students' actions and responses are recorded for subsequent analysis. The designers offer an algorithm for scoring students' problem solving. This type of tool permits both individual and large-scale assessment of student knowledge as applied to the patient problem and problem solving ability.

Standardized patients (SPs)

As a surrogate patient that can present the same patient problem to a series of students, the SP can be used to assess clinical skills, interpersonal skills, and patient education skills in a valid and acceptably reliable fashion.[56] The SP allows the exact patient problem that is needed for assessment of students to be available almost anywhere and at any time. Properly trained, the SP can give the student feedback from the patient's point of view about interpersonal and professional skills. Coming from the "patient" this can be most effective in shaping student performance in these areas. The SP is used effectively for individual student, student group, and class assessment. All of these options are described below. Over ninety percent of North American medical schools use SPs. However, the unique advantages of the SP is that they are standardized with the clinical picture and findings they present consistent between students and known to the teacher and evaluator. A specific patient problem can be chosen. Criteria for a successful performance by students can be specified ahead of time.

Students can be observed during an encounter with patients or SPs. Patients can offer physical findings that are not possible with SPs. Nevertheless, a large range of physical findings can be simulated with proper training of the SP.[57] This is an excellent assessment method for clinical skills, interpersonal skills and patient education skills for an individual student, and the assessment can be extended by an oral examination of the student. With larger numbers of students, only SPs are feasible, as it would be a fatiguing experience, and possibly damaging, for real patients to go through multiple examinations. In addition, unless properly coached (in which case they become standardized patients) real patients would not present the same findings to a series of students. A disadvantage to the observed encounter with a number of students using SPs, is the teacher time (usually clinicians) it takes to watch and assess these encounters and the concern about reliability if multiple observers are used. However, other SPs have been used to observe and score student encounters with good result.

Time in-time out is an assessment technique that can be used with standardized patients. It is useful for a real time analysis of students' application of knowledge to the patient problem and problem solving during their encounter with a patient. It can be used with the individual student or with a group of students. It is the approach used by the small group in the problem-based learning process with a SP as opposed to the PBLM and can be used for assessment. At various points in the ongoing encounter with the SP the teacher tutor, or if agreed ahead of time, the student examining the SP can call a "time out" to discuss the thinking going on at the time. During this "time out" the SP stays in role, but acts as if she or he is not in the room. In the time-out the tutor can probe the examining student's thinking (hypotheses, analysis of the patients appearance or responses, knowledge the student is bringing to bear on the problem as in the problem-based learning process) and the thinking of the other students. A discussion and evaluation of interpersonal skills of the examiner can also be made during time out. When the tutor or student announces "time in", the SP continues from the point time out was called as if nothing happened. The examining student can be rotated in the group, and the SP will act as if it is still the same examiner.

Multiple station examinations (OSCE and CPX)

In the late '70s, Ronald Harden introduced the Objective Structured Clinical Examination (OSCE) that used multiple stations each with a separate defined task for students to carry out. Students moved from station to station, very much like laboratory practicals in college. Between each station the student either answered written questions or was questioned by a teacher about the station just attended. Harden proposed this as a way to test student performance, conveniently and on a large scale with a large group or class of students. The OSCE assessed performance as opposed to the recall of facts, as at each station there was a defined performance to be carried out (interviewing a SP about headache, a child about developmental milestones, examining a patient's knee, interpreting an x-ray). Each station took only 5 to 10 minutes. The disadvantage to the OSCE is that it assesses only the ability to carry out the performance but not the students' ability to know when to carry out the performance working with a patient.

In the middle '80s the Clinical Practice Examination (CPX) was developed utilizing SPs in longer station encounters (20 to 30 minutes). It was not structured as in the OSCE. The student was only given the patient's presenting complaint (usually a chart on the examining room door) and was told to do whatever was appropriate to deal with the problem in the time available. It was called the CPX because it simulated the actual practice situation and setting. The stations are set up as examining rooms with all the usual accoutrements. The student encounters can be watched and evaluated through one-way glass and/or with a videocamera in the examining room. The CPX at Southern Illinois University involves post-encounter stations between patient stations. In these stations the students interact with a computer (a modified DxR) recording their diagnoses, patient findings, management plans for the patient, test to be ordered, etc.). They are given the results of the tests they order and asked how they effect their thinking and management. The intent of the CPX is to assess a wide range of skills; knowledge as applied to the patient, problem solving, clinical skills, interpersonal and professional skills in a way that simulates the skills and their sequence used in clinical practice. A large number of medical schools now utilize variations of the CPX .[58]

Models

There is an ever-increasing number of models that can both train and assess skills. There are models for performing such things as ophthalmoscopy, otoscopy, lumbar puncture, interpretation of heart sounds, tying sutures, etc. These can extend the range of skills that can be assessed. Computer controlled devices and virtual reality simulations now evolving will even extend this further in the future. Abrahamson and Denson with the help of aerospace engineers developed a realistic dummy "SIM I" that could be intubated and given intravenous medications.[59] The dummy could restrict and dilate, muscles fasciculate, and alter other body responses in response to the skill of the student. With faulty intubation, the dummy's teeth could be knocked out. A computer would record all the students' actions and the dummy patient's responses for subsequent analysis and feedback to the student. Unappreciated for what it had to offer that long ago ('70s), it was allowed to fall into disuse and was eventually destroyed. Imagine the patient lives and unnecessary trauma that might have been saved had it been actively used in anesthesia training for students, residents, and physicians. Recently there are similar units being designed.

Stimulated recall

This is a powerful tool that is not used enough in student assessment. It has been used as a research tool for analyzing physician reasoning.[60,61] It provides a tool to investigate in depth the knowledge, problem solving skills, clinical skills, professional and interpersonal skills of a student. The student's encounter with a SP is videotaped. As soon as the student has finished, almost before the student can reorganize his or her thinking, the student and the teacher sit down and observe a playback of the encounter. At various points the teacher can stop the tape and ask about the student's thinking, reasons for the questions or examinations performed, analysis of the data obtained from the patient, knowledge about any ideas or hypotheses expressed, impressions about the patient, comfort with the patient, and comfort about his or her performance. It is a personal diagnostic tool for assessing student performance and thinking not unlike the history and physical on the patient. Through appropriate questioning, the investigation can be taken anywhere the teacher feels is necessary to assess the student's knowledge and capabilities.

Packaging it all up

With such a wide and varied range of tools, all aspects of student performance can be assessed in ways consistent with the intents and objectives of problem-based learning and support the application of the method by students and teachers. The creative teacher can find many ways to package the assessment of students. The one important skill, central to problem-based learning, that is not assessed with any of these tools is self-directed learning. The assessment package has to be designed to assess this skill by allowing students, at some point in the assessment procedure, to determine what they need to learn and time needed for self-directed learning. The learning issues they choose and the resources they use can be recorded as well as the effectiveness of their self-directed learning in further assessing and or managing the problem.

A major concern about the use of any tool or package to assess students in problem-based learning is that it does not become teacher-centered, but remains student centered. The test cannot afford to be perceived by students as assessing the knowledge the faculty expect them to know, as opposed to what they feel they need to know. This concern can be met by faculty choosing the problems to be presented to the students in a test, and letting the students determine what they need to know to understand and competently handle the patient problem. A variety of assessment packages have been used in problem-based learning to meet all these requirements.

Triple jump

This is a package developed at McMaster University and adopted widely. Usually a basic scientist and clinician present a patient problem to students individually and assess the knowledge and skills they bring to the problem as they inquire about the patient through history and physical and laboratory tests. In this process the students are questioned by the teachers about their thinking and analysis of the problem. At the end of the session the students are asked to provide a self-evaluation, describe the learning issues they will pursue and the resources they will use. Several days later the students again meet with the teachers and the increased understanding and analysis they provide as a result of their self-directed study is assessed. This is only a brief description of what can occur in the triple jump (session one, self-directed study, and session two are the three "jumps") and many variations are possible. It consumes considerable faculty time for two teachers to meet with all the students in a group or class individually. Assessment criteria have to be carefully developed, especially if there are teams of teachers assessing, to ensure an acceptable reliability.

Progress test

This package was developed at Maastricht University and has been adopted by other problem-based learning programs. The progress test is a large collection of multiple choice questions covering all areas of the basic and clinical sciences. Although students take this test in each year of the curriculum, it is not expected that students in the first years will be able to do very well with the overall test. In each year their performance should improve and the test monitors their growth in knowledge and in what areas they may be deficient. In the later years of the curriculum it is expected that they will do quite well on the test. Over the years the test records the progress students are making as they go through the curriculum. The test is felt to preserve student-centeredness by its designers because there is too much on the test for the students to consider cramming to pass it. They are encouraged to take it without prior preparation so they can see where their strengths and weaknesses lie. The test has the advantage that it can be given to large numbers of students and easily scored. The drawback to this package is that it is unidimensional and it only assesses the recall and recognition of facts.

Performance Assessment of Self-Directed Study (PASS)

This external assessment examination for problem-based learning was designed by Kelson to complement the formal self and peer assessment performed in the tutorial group at the end of each curricular unit.[62] It takes a week to carry out. In the first part of the

PASS, each student interviews and examines three SPs who present problems that they had not encountered in the curricular unit they had just completed. Each encounter is observed and scored by a member of the clinical faculty. Students receive feedback from the observer at the end of each encounter. Each student is required to write up a complete case report on one of the patient problems they encountered and a diagnosis and treatment plan for all three. When these are turned in, the students get a description of the findings on history and physical as well as some laboratory work on each case. Because they are in the preclinical years, this puts all the students on a level playing field for the rest of the examination. They are then required to list what they think are the significant issues (basic science, clinical) in each case and indicate which of those issues they will take on as personal learning issues. After two to three days allowed for self-directed learning, the examination continues with part two of the PASS.

While a unit is underway, faculty representing the various disciplines in the unit work as a committee to provide the content for part two. They choose the SP cases to be used for part one. They decide on the basic science and clinical questions the students should be able to answer relative to each case. The members of the committee also determine what would be both an acceptable and an extended answer to these questions. Matrices for all three cases are put together for each student. They are developed for the examiners (usually tutors) to facilitate their use of the questions in the second phase of the test. These matrices contain a column with the self-directed learning issues each student chose to investigate for each case and a column with the questions listed parallel to the appropriate students' learning issues. These examining teachers also have a list of the acceptable and extended answers.

In the second phase, after self-directed study, each student is examined for 45 minutes by a tutor other than his group's own tutor. The students are asked to expound freely on the underlying mechanisms involved in each case. What ground they did not cover in that exposition is then investigated using the questions in the matrices.

As a package, this sophisticated examination assesses clinical skills, interpersonal skills, professional skills, self-directed learning skills, and the extent and quality of the students' knowledge base applied to understanding each case. It supports the problem-based learning process and is student-centered. It represents a comprehensive approach to assessment in problem-based learning. There are plans to transfer the interview approach in part two to an interactive computer program. Students feel that it is a fair test of what they are capable of doing.

Design your own

With the wide range of assessment tools that are available, the designers of a problem-based learning curriculum should be able to construct or adapt an assessment package that will give teachers and their students an accurate idea of how each student is progressing.

A chapter by Kelson "Assessment of Students for Proactive Lifelong Learning" provides the reader with a broader orientation to assessment in problem-based learning from a cognitive and historical perspective.[62] Nendaz and Tekian have carried out a literature review on assessment in problem-based learning.[63]

Chapter Sixteen

APPLYING PROBLEM-BASED LEARNING TO THE CLERKSHIP YEARS

P roblem-based learning in the preclinical years prepares students for their clerkship years where the problems they face will be real patients as they prepare for post-graduate work and eventual practice. Since problem-based learning as an authentic learning method requires medical students to carry out the sequence of behaviors expected in practice, continuity could be achieved if clerkship teaching also applies authentic problem-based learning, creating a seamless segue' into the demands of postgraduate education and subsequent practice.

In preclinical problem-based learning, the principle sources of problems for learning are patient simulations chosen to stimulate and direct student learning into appropriate content areas and to challenge the students' clinical reasoning process. Simulations allow the students' ongoing work with the patient problem to be interrupted at any point for discussion, review, reiteration or self-directed learning. The simulated problem can be left and re-entered at will. Simulations provide an educational flexibility that is essential to achieving mastery in the skills of medical practice by allowing students to practice and develop skills that will be translated to work with real patients. Real patients play a secondary role providing transfer of learning to the patient, enlarging the students' experience and knowledge base.

Augmenting patient problems in the clerkship with simulations

In the clerkship, real patients are not only the primary source of problems for learning but should be the primary source for all learning. Once students have acquired a broad enough experience with patients and their problems, information given in an occasional clinical lecture can be associated with recall of those experiences and applied in their subsequent clinical work. Unfortunately, there is a tendency in many clerkships to expose the students to all the important problems and facts in that specialty or discipline through lectures and seminars. With no solid base of clinical experiences on which to hang the clinical facts presented in the lecture, the information given has little likelihood of survival or application to practice. The clerkship, of all places in the curriculum, should be one of clinical experience, not lecture.

The motivation for lectures in the clerkship is probably due to an awareness by the teaching faculty that they have no opportunity to present the student with patients that have the problems that students should encounter during their clerkship. There are patient problems that students should experience in every clerkship. These are the common and important problems seen in every specialty. They have to be encountered, not just described in a lecture, to ensure an adequate experience for the students. This has become an even greater problem as inpatient time with patients is reduced and much of what students should experience in preparation for their careers is seen in offices and clinics pre- and post-admission.

To relieve this situation, the problem simulation formats used in preclinical problem-based learning can play a complementary but important role in clerkships to ensure that students have indeed been exposed to all the common and important patient problems. Ironically, my original stimulus for creating "problem boxes" (printed patient problem simulations) that were later used in problem-based learning[18] was to provide neurological clerks with broader experiences with neurological problems. This led to a variety of other simulation formats[19,27] all used in preclinical problem-based learning.

The use of standardized patients

These common and important problems can also be made available as standardized patients to complement what is available during the clerkship to expose the students to important patient problems. They provide a realistic way of presenting problems not available at the time on the clinical service. The students can apply their clinical skills in interview, examination and interpersonal skills. They are also important when the students' clinical skills, interpersonal skills, or ability with a special set of history taking or physical examination skills (i.e. mental status examination) are a concern.

Standardized patients also allow the clinical teacher to provide students with a "hands-on" opportunity to work with serious and emergency patient problems they could only observe during the clerkship (acute anginal pain; progressive loss of consciousness with dilating pupil; anaphylactic reaction; hypermanic behavior; hostile, combative, uncooperative patient; shock, myocardial infarction, seizures; coma; etc.). As with cockpit simulations used in aviation that can simulate dangerous, life-threatening situations in very expensive aircraft, standardized patients can provide a very real simulation of life-threatening or high risk problems with no risk either to the patient or the student.

Standardized patients can also be used early on in the clerkship as an audition to make certain students have the requisite clinical skills to be effective and focused in their patient workups and to have appropriate interpersonal skills. The standardized patient can then be used to provide the skills needed while the clinical teacher works with a small group of students using the "time-in/time-out" approach.[42] I found this an effective way to prepare second-year medical students for work in a neurological clinic where they needed to be confident in the neurological examination and were not able to take endless amounts of time working up patients. David Steward at Southern Illinois University designed a standardized patient clinic made up of patient problems that represented difficulties for clinical clerks about to work in a general internal medicine ambulatory clinic.

Standardized patients can provide a far more relevant assessment of student progress in the clerkship as they permit the faculty to see how the students can actually care for specific patient problems. The standardized patient provides a reliable standard test item of high validity that has well established its effectiveness as a clinical assessment tool.[56] This was the original use of standardized patients when the technique was first established in 1963.[64]

The facilitatory teaching skills of the clinical teacher

To translate all the objectives of preclinical, problem-based learning to clerkships, particularly the development of effective and efficient reasoning and self-directed learning skills, the clinical teachers will need to apply the facilitatory skills of the tutor (see "The Tutorial Process"). Although many clinical teachers use the popular "Socratic" approach in their clinical teaching, this is not the same as the tutors' approach in problem-based learning. Superficially they seem the same often making it difficult for clinical teachers to appreciate the difference. The Socratic approach involves questioning that is intended to bring forth from students an understanding that the teacher wants them to express. An understanding the teacher is sure should lie latent in the students' mind and would be delivered and shaped through dialectic discussion using, for example, posed statements in question form, counter examples or by carrying out a student's inappropriate answer to an absurdity. In this process, students are well aware of the teacher's opinion about the correctness of their statements and attempts to follow the teacher's thinking. Facts are frequently given by the teacher during this type of discussion and an exposition is provided for the student at the end. This is a powerful teaching method, but it is very teacher-centered and does not address the goals of problem-based learning. By contrast, in the tutorial discussion students are probed for their ideas and asked to explain or justify them and encouraged to recognize whenever they are uncertain or confused. The tutors' probing attempts to reveal student thinking and depth of understanding without allowing the student to know what the tutor thinks. The probing also attempts to allow the student to assess his or her performance and knowledge in relation to the patient problem and to recognize learning issues that need to be satisfied.

The clinical tutor can ask such things as "What do you think is going on with this patient? Why do you say that? What is your evidence? What do you think needs to be done? How adequate is your work-up of the patient (database, diagnostic ideas, treatment plans, etc.)? What are you unsure about? What do you think you need to learn? Where are you going to learn it?" The point that seems most difficult for clinical teachers to accept in applying the tutorial method is that they can ask such questions even when they do not know the answers themselves. In fact, it is healthy to admit ignorance as no one can know everything, and it is important for students to realize that everyone has to learn at any stage in their career and expertise. In problem-based learning, the student has to find the answers from other resources. However, the clinical tutor has to make decisions about the students' self-directed learning needs in the context of the pressures and activities in the clinical setting and the needs of the patient who, unlike the simulated problem, cannot be dropped at any point and returned to later. By this time in their career in medical school, the students should be able to carry out quick self-directed learning when needed. The tutor could ask. "Where will you get that information? Come back later (minutes, hours, tomorrow) and tell me what you learned and how you will revise your decisions about diagnosis or care." and in the interim make decisions about tests and treatment that have to be made to provide care. On returning to the patient or chart, the student can compare this to her or his ideas after self-study. Although self-directed learning skills need to be constantly honed, now that the students have come this far in their training, it may be appropriate on many occasions for the clinical teacher to provide the students with the information they need at the time. This should occur only after the students have identified what it is that needs to be learned and have assessed the adequacy of their performance. It would be valuable for the students to be asked to follow-up later with other resources and to check up on the clinical tutor's information.

It is important to challenge students to find the information they need at the time. This is possible if there are computerized information resources immediately available. This will become the standard required of physicians as online libraries and databases are increasingly available in clinical areas.

Continuing the small group sessions in the clerkship

Weekly small group sessions can still be carried out on the clinical services to augment the clerkship experience, and students can continue to follow the same procedure as used in problem-based learning in the preclinical years. PBLMs are just as relevant for use in the clinical years as they represent a complete patient simulation. The objectives for the small group in the preclinical years is to reason through the patient problem and learn the basic mechanisms responsible for the patient problem, the normal and abnormal form and function involved in terms of anatomy, physiology, biochemistry, behavior, pharmacology, microbiology, immunology, etc. Now in the clerkship, the groups' objectives should be the assessment (diagnosis) of the patient problem and its management in addition to the basic mechanisms responsible. In these meetings, a student can present the patient problem she or he has worked up to the group in the same manner as a PBLM. The student can provide the presenting complaint, demographic data and patient appearance. The others in the group can inquire about items on history and physical, which the presenting student will provide as with the PBLM. If the students in the group ask a question or want to perform an item of physical examination not performed on the patient by the presenting student, a discussion about why this information is important, and why the presenting student did not obtain it can occur. These requested items that were not performed should be listed, as the students might have the opportunity to visit the patient as a group subsequently and get that data. Likewise, the laboratory tests can be requested in the same manner. When the students have finished their inquiry, they should come to a conclusion about diagnosis and treatment and the justification for their decision. The presenting student, who should have researched everything he will need to know about the patient, can then provide feedback to the group about the accuracy of their assessment and appropriateness of their treatment plan as well as follow-up information concerning the patient.

Chapter Seventeen

CONVERTING TO PROBLEM-BASED LEARNING

The schools that successfully developed problem-based learning curricula have a number of factors in common. In almost all cases, the medical school dean was either a protagonist for change or made it clear to faculty interested in developing such a curriculum that he or she would provide endorsement and support for a pilot project or a curriculum in problem-based learning. The second important ingredient seems to be a dedicated group of faculty who recognize that educational change is needed and are willing to work towards developing a problem-based curriculum. The third is an effective strategy for educating faculty as a whole about problem-based learning and recruiting the interest of faculty from many different disciplines. Often a demonstration of problem-based learning by a teacher from a school with established problem-based learning, using your own students, produces wider faculty interest and support. Your faculty can see what the method is like and the students' reaction to learning in such a manner. A visit by key faculty to a problem-based learning school has a similar effect, but not as powerful as seeing your own students involved.

The first step is to determine whether or not there are enough faculty willing to be tutors, resource faculty and unit directors for the problem-based learning curriculum you want to design. Tutors and resource faculty may spend, on the average, 6 hours a week during the time of a particular unit (usually anywhere from 6 to 12 weeks in duration). The unit directors coordinate both the design of curricular units (usually organ-system units) and the design and development of problems. They need to be prepared to spend almost 50% of their time in this activity for the first year or so until the curriculum is in place and operating long enough to have all the bugs worked out. This might require negotiation with their respective chairpersons.

Although many of the earlier problem-based learning schools received outside financial support to develop their curricula, when the method was novel, it is difficult to get outside support now. The school should be willing to accept the modest costs in setting up a problem-based learning curriculum. The development of home bases, finding curriculum coordinators (scheduling, contacting, handling the necessary paperwork, and meeting needs of students and faculty), preparing faculty, creating problems, training standardized patients and preparing educational support materials need to be considered.

Problem-based learning as an alternative curriculum versus a total curriculum

Creating an alternative or problem-based learning curriculum is probably the easiest way to start in an existing, as opposed to new, medical school. Those faculty and students who would like such a curriculum can take part. Those who would not touch such a curriculum with a ten-foot pole who can avoid having anything to do with it. This is not only the easiest way, but may represent the only way a complete problem-based curriculum might be initiated. The downside is the increased demand operating a double curriculum can make on faculty and resources. New Mexico, Harvard, Bowman Gray, Rush and Southern Illinois found the parallel curriculum the only feasible way to get problem-based learning up and running in their schools. If problem-based learning is chosen for its educational advantages, then it should be available to all students. Many teachers have expressed the opinion that it is good for students to have an option in the way they learn and an alternative curriculum allows them to choose between problem-based learning and conventional learning. Since problem-based learning requires the students to develop and practice the skills and behaviors required of physicians as they learn, you might question whether those students more comfortable with lectures, being told what to learn, and taking written examinations should seriously consider a career in medicine.

For many years the only schools with a total problem-based curriculum were new schools that began that way. These were McMaster, Maastricht, and Newcastle. However, more recently, several traditional schools have totally converted to problem-based learning. Hawaii and Sherbrooke went from a conventional curriculum to a total problem-based curriculum. The basic requirements for this monumental feat seem to boil down to encouragement and support for the change from the Dean to spearhead the change, and a small group of faculty from different disciplines interested in working towards problem-based learning. Sherbrooke prefaced their conversion by putting into place a series of faculty development workshops for all faculty that gave them the skills and knowledge to undertake the change.

Curriculum Models That Do Not Work

In an attempt to try problem-based learning, often as a pilot program, many schools have undertaken models, such as the following, that have usually turned out to be unsuccessful and often frustrating, leaving a negative impression on students and faculty alike.

Problem-based learning as an add-on

When problem-based learning is added to an ongoing standard curriculum by introducing problems, tutorial sessions and self-directed learning on top of what the students already have to do, the results are very unsatisfactory. The students are not able to make a quick transition from passive learning and being told what to learn to having to problem solve, not being told what to learn, having to decide what they need to learn, digging out their own information, and then going back to the regular curriculum. They get confused as to what the rules of the game are at any particular point in the curriculum, and the teachers become exasperated having to lecture, tutor, and be resource faculty at various times. The worst aspect is that all this work is perceived as an add-on to an already taxing and demanding curriculum.

Problem-based learning as a parallel experience to a conventional curriculum

In conventional curricula, several courses are usually taught each day in parallel. If one course, say a neuroscience unit, decides it would convert totally to problem-based learning during its time, maybe from 9-12 in the mornings of each day with conventional courses running parallel, perhaps biochemistry or pharmacology in the afternoon. Confusion is reduced as both students and faculty know what is expected when in each course. The problem with this model surfaces during self-directed learning. When one medical school tried this approach in a neuroscience unit they found that during the unstructured self-directed learning time students would either be studying for snap biochemistry quizzes, preparing biochemistry laboratory reports, or reading biochemistry assignments. Conventional medical school curricula put heavy emphasis on acquiring extensive information in all subjects. Usually far more than most students feel they have time to cover. The available unstructured, self-directed learning time in a parallel problem-based learning course is gobbled up to meet the overwhelming demands of the regular curriculum.

A too short block

The problems with the foregoing models could be avoided by devoting a complete block of time to problem-based learning with no competing subjects. Such a block would provide a pilot problem-based learning curriculum. However, the blocks that are made available are often only three to four weeks in duration and new difficulties are created. Whenever a new group of students and tutors start problem-based learning, there is a tremendous amount of adjustment that is required, and characteristically everyone gets frustrated with the process and each other in about three to four weeks (see *The Tutorial Process*).[1] Once this hurdle is passed, usually all the frustrations and concerns about such things as problem solving, finding out what to learn, digging out information and getting no clear guidelines diminish, and the problem-based learning experience becomes rewarding, exciting and productive. Stopping the problem-based learning experience at three to four weeks is the wrong time and will leave the impression that problem-based learning is not rewarding or worth the effort. A block of time devoted to problem-based learning is a good way to start a pilot program, but it should run at least eight to ten weeks.

Problem-based learning in a single discipline

This can be successful if the entire course can be designed as problem-based learning. However, much of the impact of problem-based learning is lost when information from multiple disciplines involved in the problem (anatomy, physiology, behavioral, biochemical etc.) cannot be acquired and integrated around the patient problems. If there is no other way than an alternative, or parallel curriculum or an eight to ten week block it should be tried, but with the idea that if it is successful, other disciplines will be added.

Chapter Eighteen

CHOOSING PROBLEMS

The design of problem formats that present the patient problem as it is actually presented clinically and permit the student to carry out a free inquiry (asking any questions on history, performing any items of physical examination and ordering any laboratory tests in any sequence) is essential to allow the students to develop an effective and efficient clinical reasoning process. Commonly used formats to accomplish this in problem-based learning are the PBLM and standardized patient described previously and computer formats such as the DxR[43]. These problem simulations should be based on actual patients to assure students that such a problem really occurred in practice. In addition, using a real patient problem allows the problem designers to use the patient's laboratory results, x-rays, scans, pathological materials, etc. in the problem simulations.

The problems as a group are the curriculum

The problems chosen represent the curriculum in problem-based learning. Every patient problem requires the students to apply a certain body of facts and concepts to assess the problem, determine the basic mechanisms involved, and attempt resolution. If the students are ignorant, unsure, or confused about the facts and concepts required in their problem solving activity, they will recognize the need to put them on the board as learning issues and tackle them during self-directed study. In this way, problem-based learning causes them to learn and apply the facts and concepts important to their medical education. There are two ways to approach the selection of problems for a problem-based curriculum.

Two methods for selecting problems

Problem choice based on what the teacher feels should be taught

The way to select problems is based on the teachers' knowledge or belief as to what it is students ought to learn from their disciplines. This approach allows teachers to be more comfortable in the conversion from the teacher-centered, didactic learning approaches they have always used to student-centered, problem-based learning. They can be reassured through the selection of problems that stimulate the learning they feel is important that a curriculum is still intact and they are able to influence what the students should learn. However, the question can always be asked, how does the teacher in any discipline know what a medical student should learn? Physiologists may know what a graduate student needs to know in order to be a physiologist, but how do they know what a future physician needs to know? This uncomfortable question is usually sidestepped by basic science faculty with a reference to the knowledge that will be required for students to pass USMLE Step I. There is little point to challenging this, and this first approach will make them more comfortable.

In this first approach, all the disciplines in a particular curricular unit (usually in an organ system such as cardiovascular or a neuro-science) are asked to list all the concepts they feel the student should learn in that unit. For example, in a cardiovascular unit the faculty could list all the important concepts normally taught in cardiovascular physiology, anatomy, biochemistry, pharmacology, etc. as well as microbiology, immunology, pathology, behavior, etc. that might be learned in the context of the cardiovascular system. An effort should be made to eliminate all truly unnecessary, it-would-be-nice-to-know material and concentrate on what are truly the big items that are essential and relevant for student learning. This listing may be influenced by the faculty's awareness of the questions on the USMLE Step I examination, but careful decisions should be made as to what is truly essential.

Once these lists are assembled, the unit coordinator, supported by faculty as needed, can then decide on patient problems that would inevitably cause the students to have to learn concepts on the list. One patient problem will often be seen to address multiple concepts in different disciplines simultaneously. This process continues until all the listed items are checked off. Then PBLMs and standardized patient simulations can be selected or prepared. Clinical faculty can be asked to find patient records that could be used to develop appropriate problem simulations.

A matrix can be developed with the information and concepts the students are expected to learn listed down the left side of the page or computer screen vertically with horizontal ruled lines between them. The problems either proposed or designed listed horizontally across the top with vertically ruled lines between them. The items of information or concepts addressed by each problem can then be checked in the boxes that are appropriate. Since problems address multiple areas of learning, the adequacy of the problems chosen to cover the "curriculum" can be seen. Problems can then be added that will address areas not covered, and problems that repetitively cover the same areas can be modified or eliminated. The finished matrix can show other faculty or external reviewers of the curriculum how problem-based learning will meet curricular expectations

If there are concepts listed for which no patient problem can be found that will address them, then the faculty should consider whether the concepts are relevant for medical students learning in the curriculum. This question can also be considered if only an extremely rare and unusual patient problem would address a concept on the list.

In choosing these patient problems, it is important to choose problems that are common or prevalent as well as problems that, although not common, should be recognized and managed because of their high morbidity or mortality. This thinking leads to the second, more relevant way, for choosing problems.

Selecting problems by prevalence and impact

The other approach to the selection of problems for a curricular unit, such as a cardiovascular unit, would be to choose those cardiovascular problems that are common and likely to be encountered by the student no matter what field of medicine he or she might pursue. Problems that are important because of their potential impact on the patient, and those that may represent an important model for a group of diseases. MacDonald has a formula for problem selection at McMaster Medical School based on a number of criteria including magnitude, severity, effectiveness of intervention, and treatability.[65] You can then decide that whatever it is that students need to learn to understand the basic mechanisms involved in these problems should determine the curriculum. This approach is uncomfortable for many faculty initially, especially those concerned about the students scores on the USMLE. However, it ensures that the curriculum is relevant and up-to-date for the education of physicians. Periodic review of all problems and the addition of new ones that reflect new information, diseases, treatments, diagnostic tests or changes in disease prevalence that have surfaced will automatically keep learning in the curriculum relevant.

As mentioned initially, it is important that real patient problems are used in problem-based learning so that students can always be reassured that the problem really occurred and you can use laboratory tests and other patient materials in assembling the problem. However, it is often necessary to "tune" them to take advantage of the potential that a particular problem might have to stress an important concept. They often need to be tuned to highlight ethical, legal, psychosocial, nutritional or epidemiological concepts, as only a few examples.

It is also important to have faculty from different disciplines and content areas to periodically review the problems in a unit to see if concepts, particularly new concepts in their discipline, are being addressed.

Chapter Nineteen

EVALUATING THE EFFECTIVENESS OF PROBLEM-BASED LEARNING AS AN INSTRUCTIONAL METHOD

The Josiah Macy Jr. Foundation sponsored a conference in 1989 to consider how innovative curricula should be evaluated to determine if there are distinctively different outcomes from traditional curricula. The conference concentrated on problem-based and community-oriented curricula, and the report of that conference by Friedman et al. provides a very thoughtful analysis of what should be evaluated, where differences might be expected, and what should not be evaluated as differences would probably not be significant.[66] They listed 26 areas where differences might be expected and five where no differences might be expected. The latter list concerned passing rates on licensing and certification examinations, likelihood of making a major clinical mistake in practice, clinical problem solving with common and uncomplicated conditions, educational costs per student (after start-up costs), and the cost efficiency of graduates. They offered specific recommendations for evaluating five outcomes that are felt to be important: psychosocial and inter-personal skills, continuing learning, satisfaction, clinical problem solving, and the cost of education (they expect no differences in the last two). This is an interesting resource for all schools to consider if they have problem-based curricula or plan to develop one.

Recently, four papers have been published that attempted to summarize the results of published research on the effectiveness of problem-based learning.[9,10,11] Two apply meta-analyses to the available published data each felt was appropriate to use in analyzing and judging the outcomes of problem-based learning. They both are rich in data and references. Albanese and Mitchell state in their meta-analysis that they "attempted to maintain an objective, if not somewhat skeptical posture." This posture has caused them to make some generalizations from some studies with inadequate data or data of questionable significance. Their paper is valuable if carefully read, and if in each section dealing with a different outcome, the reader reviews their data, and then draws his or her own conclusion first, and then compares it to the authors'.

The paper by Vernon and Blake used different criteria for the papers they included in their meta-analysis, and it contains more recent references. Vernon and Blake compared their meta-analysis with Albanese and Mitchell's and noted that they had similar conclusions. Both found student satisfaction and clinical performance to favor problem-based learning. Vernon and Blake found the difference to be significant. Both meta-analyses found an increase in clinical knowledge as determined by tests, but the difference was not significant. Both studies indicated greater faculty satisfaction with problem-based learning, and both studies suggested that students in problem-based learning had greater strengths in self-directed learning and tended to learn by understanding as opposed to rote memorization, although the available information was scanty. The recent study by Regan-Smith, Small, et al.[48] provides richer data involving six medical schools and shows a significant difference between students in a problem-based curriculum and in a traditional curriculum. Students in problem-based learning learn principally by understanding as opposed to traditional students who learn primarily by memorizing without understanding.

As there are so many different educational methods that are all called problem-based learning, attempts at meta-analysis are weakened as a technique for pooling studies, inadequate in themselves due to limited subjects or dissimilar curricula, to obtain more analytic power. A meta-analysis assumes that all studies are based on the same method. Nevertheless, both studies were carefully and thoughtfully performed and provide a treasure for any teachers interested in what all the presently available research data may show about problem-based learning. Vernon and Blake conclude that "The present meta-analysis of evaluative research indicates that it is unlikely that students will suffer detrimental consequences from exposure to PBL programs. Our analysis suggests some educational benefits from PBL in comparison with more traditional approaches. The analysis highlights the need for methodological rigorous studies that further address the value and effects of PBL."[10]

Dick Mårtenson, an educator at the Karolinska Institute, asked the question, "Is problem-based learning beneficial?" and provided a research overview. This review contrasts with the meta-analyses as it represents the opinion of an experienced educator who has looked at selected research he felt was significant. His conclusions are that "Students in PBL do not learn less and that they seem to enjoy their program very much." He comments that "The characteristics of PBL and the focus of the teachers involved are in accordance with research findings in learning psychology." Further, he adds, "The way students work in PBL seems to reflect the way clinicians think and work when they solve clinical problems as well as the way researchers approach their tasks."[67]

A paper by Susan Williams puts problem-based learning into the context of other well established learning methods used outside of medicine that have features in common with problem-based learning.[68] She discusses a number of newer instructional methods that put the learner in the real world context such as cognitive apprenticeship developed by Collins and his group and Anchored Instruction developed by Bransford's group that have educational aims quite similar to problem-based learning. She then carries out an analysis of case-based instruction as used in law and problem-based learning in medicine. This is a useful paper for teachers wanting the view of an educator outside of medicine.

The most valuable assessments of PBL are longitudinal studies that measure outcomes in terms of physician performance in the real world of practice after completion of formal medical educational training. Are they more effective and efficient clinicians? Do they remain informed and contemporary in their practice by virtue of self-directed learning skills? Are they more effective in medical care teams? Do they apply problem-based learning in their own educational tasks? Data needed for longitudinal assessment are, however, difficult to obtain, and only a few studies have been carried out.

The studies coming out of McMaster based on data from Ontario's provincial practice plan, now that their graduates are out in practice in greater numbers, will be of increasing interest.[69,70] The present information is limited but suggests that there is a measurable difference in the McMaster graduate. McMaster produces a higher percentage of physicians entering primary care medicine than other graduates of Canadian schools. They also have produced a greater number of physicians who have gone into academic or research pursuits. Spending about the same amount of time in practice, they see fewer patients, earn less, and provide more psychotherapy in their practice. What of these outcomes relate to their education or other factors also unique to McMaster, such as their admission policy, has yet to be determined. Hopefully, more data will come from other sources that may provide answers concerning other questions described before. In a few years other problem-based schools will have the opportunity to track their products into practice, and I hope they take full advantage of the situation. Agreeing to follow-up assessments through residency, and later into practice, should be an admission requirement of all students entering a problem-based learning curriculum.

As mentioned in the introduction, most faculty undertake problem-based learning because the method makes sense to them. The fact that students are treated like adults responsible for their own learning and empowered to think and dig out facts on their own are the behaviors desired in the physician-to-be. To faculty working in both problem-based and regular curricula, problem-based learning seems to produce a different student. Their enthusiasm for learning and the more collegial relationship they have with faculty teachers are positive for both students and faculty. The faculty get to know students better than with any other teaching method. The students work with the faculty to constantly improve the curriculum and often take on curricular responsibilities themselves. The information they discover on self-directed learning can be a learning experience for the faculty. The bottom-line for many faculty in problem-based learning is that they enjoy teaching in this manner and the students enjoy learning in this way. This is clearly shown in both meta-analyses and Mårtenson's paper.

More recent studies have indicated the effectiveness of problem-based learning. Distlehorst and Robbs compared the performance of students in the parallel preclinical problem-based learning curriculum at Southern Illinois University (SIU) with the students in the standard curriculum for a period of four years.[71] The problem-based learning curriculum at SIU, analyzed in this study, is an authentic problem-based learning curriculum meeting all the requirements listed in this book. The scores obtained by the students in the United States Medical Licensing Examination (USMLE) in both curricula and their performance in the clinical clerkship were compared. There was no significant difference seen in the

USMLE scores suggesting that the problem-based learning curriculum did no harm in terms of facts learned as measured by the USMLE. The student performance scores that were studied in the clerkships were provided by clinical faculty who were generally unaware of which preclinical curriculum any of the clerkship students attended, and the competencies evaluated are the same as those evaluated for many years. The problem-based learning students mean scores were higher and the difference was significant overall as well as for several of the individual clerkships. This performance difference held across the entire clerkship year for these students. Richards, Ober, et al carried out a similar study comparing the performance of students in a parallel preclinical problem-based learning curriculum with those in the conventional curriculum at Bowman Gray Medical School. While the study was limited to the performance of students in an Internal Medicine clerkship, it produced essentially the same results.[72]

Shinn, Haynes, et al. compared practicing physicians who were graduates of McMaster University, a total problem-based learning curriculum throughout its three years, with graduates of the University of Toronto, when there was no problem-based learning curriculum in place.[73] They assessed how well these graduates, now in practice five years or more, kept abreast of the changes that occurred in the care of hypertension. The McMaster graduates were significantly better informed, suggesting that the emphasis on developing skills in self-directed learning in problem-based learning curricula was effective.

The performance of graduates once out in practice is the key to confirming the advantages of problem-based learning for those who need to be convinced. Studies that measure their performance (what they do, not what they know) in terms of patient care are needed to truly address the putative outcomes for problem-based learning. This is not easy, but needs to be done.

Chapter Twenty

CRITERIA FOR ANALYZING
A PROBLEM-BASED LEARNING CURRICULUM

In the beginning of this book, the difficulty in generalizing about problem-based learning from the reports and studies of individual schools that claim to use problem-based learning was described. Most medical teachers are unaware of the many marked differences that can be present in these schools. Teachers in a problem-based curriculum may be unaware of how unique their own curriculum might actually be. Because of this, it is erroneous to generalize about problem-based learning from observations or reports from a particular school without fully understanding the method actually used. To more fully understand a particular problem-based learning method the following list is offered. It should help you to more carefully characterize and evaluate any particular problem-based learning curriculum you may hear or read about, or have a chance to visit. Also, it is important for those describing their problem-based learning curriculum to consider describing these variables in their descriptions. These criteria are based on the discussions of problem-based learning in this book.

1) Over what span of time does the problem-based learning curriculum occur (weeks, months, one or more years, the entire curriculum)?

2) Is the problem-based experience designed for all students or for a subset (alternative or parallel curriculum)?

3) How is the time for problem-based learning distributed over the calendar (several hours each day, one day a week, several days a week, or full-time for a unit, block, semester, course, year or more)?

4) Is the problem-based experience an add-on to the regular curriculum without modification or reduction of what students have always had to learn in the regular curriculum?

5) How many subjects are integrated into the problem-based learning experience for the students (occurs within only one subject, multiple subjects are integrated, all but one subject, all subjects are integrated)?

6) What subjects are taught outside of problem-based learning, and what methods are used to teach those subjects?

7) If problem-based learning occurs throughout a block, course, year, are there other teaching/learning methods used outside of the problem-based experience (lectures, laboratories)? If there are other teaching/learning methods, are they integrated into the problem-based learning curriculum? Are they optional for the student to take or attend?

8) Is the problem-based learning experience designed for small groups of students or the whole class?

9) If it is designed for small groups, how many students are in the group?

10) Are one or two tutors used? If more than one is used what are their respective roles?

11) What is the background of the tutors (basic scientists, clinicians, senior students, educators, nurses, etc.)?

12) What kind of training is used to prepare the tutors?

13) How are tutors evaluated and by whom?

14) Which of the following stages in the problem-based learning process are used by tutors?
   a) Reasoning through the problem using the hypothetico-deductive process.
   b) Identification of learning issues.
   c) Identification of information resources to be employed during self-directed learning.
   d) Critique of learning resources on return from self-study.
   e) Application of newly acquired information back to the problem.
   f) Discussion of learning to achieve integration, abstraction, and transfer.
   g) Self-assessment by students.
   h) Peer assessment by students.

15) How are problems designed (are they well-structured case histories, case vignettes or ill-structured)?

16) Do the problem simulation formats used permit students to freely inquire about findings on history, physical and laboratory tests?

17) Are there experiences with standardized patients and real patients incorporated into the problem-based learning experience?

18) What is the role of resource faculty or other teaching faculty outside of the tutor? Do they respond to the students' learning needs (student-centered) or do they provide faculty-determined information to students (faculty centered)?

19) How are students assessed? This is such a powerful influence on the way students will study and on how student-centered the curriculum is, that the methods used should be carefully characterized.

20) Are they given grades or pass/fail scores and how are these determined?

These questions may not be sufficient in themselves to determine how independent students are in their learning (how student-centered the curriculum method employed). There are so many subtle ways that faculty can prescribe what should be learned as opposed to providing guidance to students as they make their own learning decisions. The curriculum may have to be observed in action.

The answers to these questions can help you determine how well any particular problem-based curriculum meets all the educational objectives possible. They serve only as a basis for your own analysis of problem-based curriculum and may be insensitive to the unique design of a particular curriculum and will need to be modified.

A recent study by Kelson and Distlehorst surveyed North American medical schools about their use of problem-based learning in their curriculum. Of the 124 schools that were asked by questionnaire if they used problem-based learning 85 indicated they had some sort of problem-based learning going on in their school. A more detailed questionnaire was then sent asking for details about their use of problem-based learning. They asked for many details similar to the items listed above with an emphasis on the use of groups and assessment. They concluded that problem-based learning has become a generic category that involves almost any teaching approach. They note that despite this wide variability that almost all the schools expected the full range of student outcomes for problem-based learning; knowledge, problem solving, self-directed learning and collaboration. "It is almost as if the problem-based learning label itself is meant to magically confer results." They discuss how the process in the authentic problem-based learning model described here models the projected outcomes for problem-based learning, and combined with the group process works towards producing these outcomes. This is a valuable study that can profitably be reviewed by those who would like to see how widely problem-based learning is applied and how these variations should affect any outcomes expected for the method.

APPENDIX I

OBJECTIVES FOR UNIT 10
NERVOUS SYSTEM, MUSCULOSKELETAL SYSTEM AND PSYCHIATRY
Southern Illinois University School of Medicine
Problem-Based Learning Curriculum

A) Development of Effective and Efficient Clinical Reasoning Skills

When you encounter a patient (simulated patient, real patient, or PBLM) and have been presented with the patient's chief complaint you should be able to:

1) Generate a number of hypotheses to explain the patient's problem. These hypotheses should refer to anatomical locations, pathophysiological (or disease) processes, psychophysiological process, etiological mechanisms down to the organ, tissue, cellular, or molecular level as appropriate to guide investigation into the patient's problem.

2) Through a focused (deductive) inquiry (history and physical examination) obtain information needed to determine the correct hypothesis(es).
   a) you should be able to perform the interview and physical examination techniques required.
   b) when you are working with a patient or standardized patient, you should employ appropriate interpersonal and communication skills.

3) Analyze the data obtained from the patient in the light of the hypotheses considered, in terms of the basic mechanisms responsible for all symptoms and signs and laboratory findings.

4) Synthesize the significant data acquired in this inquiry/analysis process into an organized, developing picture of the patient's problem.
   a) this synthesis should be in terms of pathophysiological (pathological, immunological, microbiological) or psychophysiological mechanisms at the appropriate level (organ, tissue, cellular, molecular).
   b) the organization should be in a cause and effect scenario if possible to describe the chain of events, processes and structures involved.

5) Review hypotheses, inquiry, and synthesis as you progress in your problem solving process and as new information, or lack of helpful information, may dictate.

6) Choose appropriate laboratory or diagnostic procedures to either substantiate the hypothesis(es) considered to better determine the pathophysiological or psychopathological processes involved.

7) As the results of these tests and procedures become known, continue with the analysis and synthesis described above.

8) Design an appropriate pharmacological intervention, if appropriate or possible.

9) Determine what epidemiological, patient care, health care, moral or ethical issues might be involved in the diagnosis or treatment of this patient.

B) Development of Effective and Efficient Self-Directed Study Skills.

During the problem solving process with the patient problem the student should be able to recognize when more knowledge is needed to better define and understand the pathophysiological or psychophysiological mechanisms responsible for the patient problem and how they might be managed (this includes both the mechanisms involved in the patient problems in this unit and facts and related concepts that are germane to the basic science disciplines involved).

1) The most appropriate resources for obtaining this new information should be determined and appropriately used. There should be an emphasis on:
   a) faculty as resource consultants
   b) primary sources of information from the library.

2) The accuracy, adequacy and timeliness of resources should be critiqued.

3) The new knowledge acquired should be applied to the evaluation and management of the patient's problem. And prior knowledge and reasoning used with the problem should be critiqued.

C) The Depth and Focus of the Knowledge Acquired in this Learning Process

Using the reasoning and self-directed process outlined above, the students should be able to analyze the pathophysiology of the patient's problem down to the organ, tissue, cellular and subcellular level, if possible. The normal form and function (anatomy, physiology of the patient's problem down to the organ, tissue, cellular and subcellular level, if possible. The normal form and function (anatomy, physiology, behavior) of the structures and processes involved should also be understood.

D) Development of Conceptual Skills

The new knowledge acquired during work with each patient problem should be organized into an overall understanding of the nervous system and musculoskeletal system. The dynamics of disease processes and concept that are important in understanding future problems that will be encountered in these systems should be considered. Newly acquired knowledge should be reviewed in the light of related problems considered in the past to see if larger principles or rules of thumb can be derived.

E) Development of Team Skills

Each student should contribute to and support the group in its tasks with patient problems by:

1) Actively contributing to the group problem solving process.

2) Learning from and accepting help from others in the group.

3) Teaching and helping others in the group as appropriate in the learning process.

4) Accepting constructive criticism from others in the group.

5) Providing constructive criticism to others.

6) Taking responsibility for tasks required in the group's ongoing work.

7) Working with others in the self-directed learning. This includes preparing notes, diagrams, outlines, and bringing in materials that would contribute to the work of the group and the learning of others.

APPENDIX II

THE PROBLEM-BASED LEARNING MODULE (PBLM)

The PBLM is a patient simulation in book format based on an actual patient case. It is designed to allow the student to ask any question on history and perform any item of physical examination in any sequence desired. With each question the student learns the patient's answer, often in the patient's own words. With each item of the physical examination performed, the student learns what would be observed with the actual patient. In a similar manner, the student can order any laboratory tests and diagnostic investigation and discover what results would be found with the patient. In summary, almost anything that can be done with the actual patient in the clinical setting on workup can be done with this simulation.

If the information asked for was not actually obtained from the real patient, the case author creates the probable response that would have been obtained based on knowledge of the patient and the patient's illness. Also, students never get a response such as "normal" or "unremarkable." Instead they always get the actual response or finding and have to judge whether it is normal or unremarkable. As with real patients students can explore the wrong path in working up the patient or do a brilliant relevant workup.

Another section of the PBLM will allow the student to follow the progress of the actual patient as cared for by those involved with the patient at the time. If desired, it is easy for the students to receive the results of the laboratory tests requested during their initial workup in the time those results would normally come back during the ongoing care of the patient as they are following the patient's progress.

Structure of the PBLM

This simulation in book form is accomplished by:

1) An opening page describing the patient's initial complaint and the health setting in which the patient is encountered. There is usually a picture of the patient (this may not be the actual

patient, but someone that shows the appearances of the actual patient).

2) A "Master Action List" that lists all the questions, items of physical examination, laboratory and diagnostic tests that might be performed on any patient with any problem in logical, grouped, alphabetized sequence that facilitates their being easily found. Each action has a symbol (Q for question, E for examination item, T for test) and a number. This list is the same for all PBLMs and is available in a small companion booklet that can be used with any PBLM, called the "User's Guide." This guide also suggests various ways the PBLM can be used in different educational settings and with varying educational goals.

3) A history section, physical examination section and laboratory test section are all bound in the PBLM with dividers. Each section has numbered pages that provide the response to the numbers in the Master Action List.

The PBLM contains additional materials that provide feedback to the student about their performance with the problem:

4) A data sheet that contains all the important elements in the problem as a guide to faculty in their selection and use of the problem. This is not looked at by the students.

5) Reproductions of imaging, x-rays, electrocardiograms, funduscopic pictures, as appropriate, for students to study. The findings on these items are on a separate page allowing the students to first interpret them themselves.

Procedure

After reading the initial complaint of the patient, the students can decide what questions they would like to ask, find the question in the Master Action List (in the User's Guide or PBLM itself), turn to the appropriate page and learn the patient's answer. In this manner the workup can continue through history and physical. In the problem-based learning group with the tutor, the students will be recording their hypotheses on a chalkboard or equivalent, recording the significant findings they feel they have obtained, and noting learning issues as described in Chapters Nine and Ten. Once they have completed their workup they can decide on the tests that should be ordered and the management undertaken. Later, they can follow the course of the actual patient and find the results of the tests they ordered when they would be reported during the patient's progress.

A list of PBLMs can be found on <http://www.pbli.org>.

REFERENCES

[1] Barrows HS. *The Tutorial Process*, Southern Illinois University School of Medicine, Springfield, Illinois, 1988.

[2] Spaulding WB. *Revitalizing Medical Education*. BC Decker Inc., Philadelphia, Hamilton (Canada). 1991.

[3] Neufeld VR and Barrows HS. The "McMaster philosophy": An approach to medical education. *Journal of Medical Education*, 49(11): 1040-50, 1974.

[4] Kaufman A. *Lessons from Successful Innovations: Implementing Problem-Based Medical Education*. Springer Publishing Co., New York. 1985.

[5] Kantrowitz MP, Kaufman A, Mennin S, Fulop T and Guilbert J. An experimental approach to change relevant to health needs. *Innovative Tracks at Established Institutions for the Education of Health Personnel*. Geneva: World Health Organization (WHO) Offset Publication 0303-7878: 101, 1987.

[6] Anderson AS. Conversion to problem-based learning in 15 months. in *The Challenge of Problem-based Learning*. Boud D and Feletti G. Eds. Kogan Page, London. 1991.

[7] Des Marchais JE, Bureau MA, Dumais B and Pigeons G. From traditional to problem-based learning: A case report of complete curricular reform. *Medical Education*, 26: 190-199,1992.

[8] *AAMC Curriculum Directory* 1991. 20th Edition (chart supplement). Association of American Medical Colleges. Washington DC. 1992

[9] Albanese MA and Mitchell S. Problem-based learning: a review of literature on its outcomes and implementation issues. *Academic Medicine*, 68(1): 52-81, 1993

[10] Vernon DT and Blake RL. Does problem-based learning work? A meta-analysis of evaluative research. *Academic Medicine*, 68(7): 550-63, 1993.

[11] Berkson L. Problem-based learning: Have the expectations been met? *Academic Medicine*, 68: S79-88 (October supplement), 1993.

[12] Woodward CA. The effects of the innovations in medical education at McMaster: A report on follow-up studies. *MEDUCS* (Switzerland), 2: 64-68, 1989.

[13] Dornhorst AC. Information overload: Why medical education needs a shake-up. *Lancet*, 2(8245): 513 - 514, 1981.

[14] Kelson ACM and Distlehorst LH. Groups in problem-based learning (PBL): Essential elements in theory and practice. In Everson DH and Hmelo CE (Eds.) *Problem-Based Learning: A Research Perspective on Learning Interactions*. Lawrence Erlbaum Associates, New Jersey. 167-184, 2000.

[15] Norman GR and Schmidt HG. The psychological basis of problem-based learning: A review of the evidence. *Academic Medicine*, 67(9): 557-65, 1992.

[16] Schmidt HG. Foundations of problem-based learning: Some explanatory notes. *Medical Education*, 27:422-32, 1993.

[17] Myers A. Cognitive science insights for professions' education. *Journal of Optometric Education*, 15(4): 105-110, 1990.

[18] Barrows HS and Mitchell DL. An innovative course in undergraduate neuroscience: Experiment in problem-based learning with "problem boxes." *British Journal of Medical Education*, 9(4): 223-30, 1975.

[19] Barrows HS and Tamblyn RM. The portable patient problem pack: A problem-based learning unit. *Journal of Medical Education*, 52(12): 1002-4, 1977.

[20] Barrows HS and Tamblyn RM. *Guide to the developement of skills in problem-based learning and clinical (diagnostic) reasoning.* Project for Learning Resources Design (PLRD) monograph #1. McMaster University, Faculty of Medicine, Hamilton. 1976.

[21] Barrows HS and Tamblyn RM. *Problem-based learning in health sciences education.* Contract No 1 LM-6-4721, US Department of Health, Education and Welfare, Public Health Service, National Institutes of Health, National Library of Medicine, National Medical Audiovisual Center. 1979.

[22] Barrows HS and Tamblyn RM. An evaluation of problem-based learning in small groups utilizing a simulated patient. *Journal of Medical Education*, 51(1): 52-4, 1976.

[23] Barrows HS and Tamblyn RM. *Problem-Based Learning: An Approach to Medical Education*, Springer Publishing Company, New York. 1980.

[24] Barrows HS, Tamblyn RM, Gliva G, Baxter D, Murray J and Dunne P. Design and evaluation of problem-based learning units in neurology. *Transactions, American Neurological Association*, 104: 236-8, 1979.

[25] Tamblyn RM, Barrows HS and Gliva G. An initial evaluation of learning units to facilitate problem-solving and self-directed study (portable patient problem pack). *Medical Education*, 14: 394-400, 1980.

[26] Barrows H, Tamblyn R and Jenkins M. Preparing faculty for inovative educational roles. *Journal of Medical Education*, 51: 592-4, 1976.

[27] Distlehorst LH and Barrows HS. A new tool for problem-based self-directed learning. *Journal of Medical Education*, 57(6): 486-8, 1982.

[28] Barrows HS. *How to Design a Problem-Based Curriculum for Preclinical Years*. Springer Publishing Company, New York. 1985.

[29] Loschen EL. Student-centered, teacher guided medical education. Presented at the Maastricht University 20th Anniversary Conference *Placing the Student at the Centre: Current implementations of student-centered education.* November, 1996.

[30] Barrows HS and Pickell GC. *Developing Clinical Problem-Solving Skills: A Guide to More Effective Dagnosis and Treatment.* Norton Medical Books, W.W. Norton & Co, New York, London, 1991.

[31] Barrows HS and Feltovich PJ. The clinical reasoning process. *Medical Education,* 21(2):86-91, 1987.

[32] Elstein AS, Shulman LS and Sprafka SS. *Medical Problem-Solving: An Analysis of Clinical Reasoning.* Harvard University Press, Cambridge, MA and London. 1978.

[33] Barrows HS, Norman GR, Neufeld VR and Feightner JW. The clinical reasoning of randomly selected physicians in general medical practice. *Clinical and Investigative Medicine - Medecine Clinique et Experimentals,* 5(1):49-55, 1982.

[34] Gale J and Marsden P. *Medical Diagnosis: From Student to Clinician.* Oxford University Press, London. 1983.

[35] Gilhooly KJ. Cognitive psychology and medical diagnosis. *Applied Cognitive Psychology,* 4: 261-272, 1990.

[36] Feltovich P, Johnson PE, Moller JH and Swanson DB. The role and development of medical knowledge in diagnostic expertise. In Clancey WJ. Shortliffe E. *Readings in Medical Artificial Intelligence: The First Decade.* Addison Wesley, Reading MA, 1984.

[37] Feltovich PJ and Barrows HS. Issues of generality in medical problem solving. In Schmidt HG and DeVolder ML.(Eds.), *Tutorials in Problem-Based Learning: New Directions in Training for the Health Professions.* Van Gorcum, Assen/Maastricht, The Netherlands, 1984.

[38] Schmidt HG, Norman JR and Boshuizen HPA. A cognitive perspective on medical expertise: Theory and implications. *Academic Medicine,* 65(10): 611-621, 1990.

[39] Medawar PB. *Introduction and Intuition in Scientific Thought.* Metheun, London. 1969.

[40] Chamberlain TC. The method of multiple working hypotheses. (Reprinted from Science 1890;15:92). *Science,* 148(5): 754-9, 1965.

[41] Sagan C. *Broca's Brain.* Ballantine Books, New York, 1980.

[42] Barrows HS. *Simulated (standardized) Patients and Other Human Simulations.* Health Sciences Consortium, Chapel Hill, NC. 1988.

[43] Myers JH., Dorsey JK and Benz E. *Diagnostic Reasoning (DxR)* Author Manual. Carbondale IL 1993.

[44] Squire LR. Mechanisms of memory. *Science*, 232: 1612-19, 1986.

[45] Schon DA. *The Refletive Practitioner.* Basic Books Inc., New York, 1983.

[46] Levine HG and Forman PM. A study of retention of knowledge of neurosciences information. *Journal of Medical Education*, 48(9): 867-69, 1973.

[47] Baddeley AD. Domains of recollection. *Psychological Review*, 89: 708-29, 1982.

[48] Regan-Smith M, Small Jr. P, Obenshain SS, Zeitz H, Richards B and Woodward C. *Student learning through rote memorization in traditional compared to problem-based schools: Is it different?* Paper and abstract presented to the Research in Medical Education conference (p45), Annual meeting of the American Association of Medical Colleges, Washington DC., November 1993.

[49] Sackett DL and Haynes RB. *Determinants of the decision to treat.* Presentation to the Society for Epidemiological Research, Toronto Canada, June 15-18, 1976.

[50] Ramsey PG, Carline JD, Inui TS, Larson EB, LoGerfo JP, Noricini JJ and Wenrich MD. Changes over time in the knowledge base of practicing internists. *JAMA*, 266(8); 1103-7, 1991.

[51] Sackett DL, Richardson WS, Rosenberg W and Haynes RB. *Evidence Based Medicine: How to Practice and Teach EBM.* New York, Churchill Livingstone, 1997.

[52] Barrows HS. A taxonomy of problem-based learning methods. *Medical Education*, 20: 481-486,1986.

[53] Rankin JA. Problem-based medical education: Effect on library use. *Bull Med Libr Assoc*, 80(1): 36-43, 1992.

[54] Szekely L. Productive processes in learning and thinking. *Acta Psychologica*, 7: 388-407, 1950.

[55] Spiro RJ, Coulson RL, Feltovich PJ and Anderson DK. Cognitive flexibility theory: Advanced knowledge acquisition in ill-structured domains. *Proceedings of the 10th annual conference of the cognitive science society.* Lawrence Erlbaum Assoc., Hillsdale NJ, 1988.

[56] Proceedings of the AAMC's Consensus Conference on the use of standardized patients in the teaching and evaluation of clinical skills. *Academic Medicine*, 68(6): 437-483, 1993.

[57] Barrows HS. *Training Standardized Patients to have Physical Findings.* Southern Illinois University School of Medicine, Springfield, IL. 1999.

[58] Morrison LJ and Barrows HS. *Educational Impact of the Macy Consortia: Regional Development of Clinical Practice Examinations.* Southern Illinois University School of Medicine, Springfield, IL, 1998.

[59] Abrahamson S, Denson JS and Wolf R. Effectiveness of a simulator in training anesthesia residents. *Journal of Medical Education.* 44(6): 515-519, 1969.

[60] Barrows HS, Norman GR, Neufeld VR and Feightner JW. The clinical reasoning of randomly selected physicians in general medical practice. *Clinical Investigative Medicine.* 1982;5(1): 49-55.

[61] Elstein AS, Shulman LS and Sprafka SS. *An Analysis of Medcical Inquiry Process.* Cambridge, MA. Harvard University Press. 1978.

[62] Kelson ACM. Epilogue: Assessment of Students for Proactive Lifelong Learning. In Everson DH and Hmelo CE (Eds.) *Problem-Based Learning: A Research Perspective on Learning Interactions.* Lawrence Erlbaum Associates, New Jersey. 315-345, 2000.

[63] Nandaz MR and Tekian A. Assessment in problem-based learning medical schools: A literature review. *Teaching and Learning in Medicine,* 11(4):232-243. 1999.

[64] Barrows HS and Abrahamson S. The programmed patient: A technique for appraising student performance in clinical neurology. *Journal of Medical Education,* 39(8): 802-4, 1964.

[65] MacDonald PJ. Selection of health problems for a problem-based curriculum. In Boud D and Feletti G. (Eds.) *The Challenge of Problem-Based Learning.* Kogan Page, London. 1991.

[66] Friedman CP, de Bliek R, Greer DS, Mennin SP, Norman GR, Sheps CG, Swanson DB and Woodward CA. Charting the winds of change: Evaluating innovative medical curricula. *Academic Medicine,* 65: 8-14, 1990.

[67] Mårtenson D. Is problem-based learning beneficial? A research overview. *Educao Médica,* 4: 2-9, 1993.

[68] Williams SM. Putting case-based instruction into context: Examples from legal and medical education. *Journal of the Learning Sciences,* 2(4): 367-427, 1992.

[69] Woodward CA. The effects of the innovations in medical education at McMaster: a report on follow-up studies. *MEDUCS* (Switzerland), 2(3): 64-68, 1989.

[70] Woodward CA. Monitoring an innovation in medical education: The McMaster experience. In Nooman EZ, Schmidt HG, and Ezzat ES. (Eds.) *Innovations in Medical Education: And Evaluation of its Present Status.* Springer Publishing, New York. 1990.

[71] Distlehorst LH and Robbs RS. A comparison of problem-based learning and standard curriculum students: Three years of retrospective data. *Teaching and Learning in Medicine*,10(3): 131-137, 1998.

[72] Richards BF, Ober KP, Cariaga-Lo L, Camp MG, Philp J, McFarlane M, Rupp R and Zaccaro DJ. Ratings of students' performances in a third-year internal medicine clerkship: A comparison between problem-based and lecture-based curricula. *Academic Medicine* 71(2):187-189. February 1996.

[73] Shin JH, Haynes RB and Johnston ME. Effect of problem-based, self-directed undergraduate education on life-long learning. *Canadian Medical Association Journal.* 148(6), 969-976, 1993.

INDEX

Alternative (parallel) versus total PBL curricula, 93, 118-119

Assessment of students in PBL, 36, 98-110

Authentic PBL, 37-47

Authenticity of PBL, 81-84

Changing to PBL (see convert ing to PBL), 85, 87, 91, 118

Clerkships, using PBL in, x, 1, 111-116

Climate and roles, 49

Clinical experience in PBL, 46, 78, :12

Clinical practice simulated by PBL, 3, 22, 82-84

Clinical reasoning process, 12-22, 91

Cognitive flexibility, 73

Commitment, 62

Concerns of medical teachers about PBL, 85-89

Converting to PBL, 117-121

Criteria for analyzing a PBL curriculum, 130-133

Curricular models of PBL that will not work, 119

Curricular requirements for authentic PBL, 37-47

Data analysis in PBL process, 16

Data synthesis, 16

Diagnostic and treatment decisions, 17

Discipline consultants, 44, 86

Evaluating the effectiveness of PBL, 125-129

Evaluation of different PBL methods, 130-133

First session with a new problem, 51

Goals of undergraduate medical education, 4-6

Goals for PBL (see objectives for PBL)

Grades versus pass/fail, xii, 76, 92, 98

Home base, 66, 118

Hypotheses, generation of, 13-14

Illness script, 16

Individual as opposed to group learning, 77

Inefficiency of traditional teaching methods, 28

Inquiry strategy, 14-15

Integrating other learning methods into PBL, 89-90

Introductions in the small group, 49

Knowledge, its relation to the clinical reasoning process, 13, 23-29

Learning issues review, 62

Learning resources, 45, 65

Learning sequence in PBL, 48-81, 84

Learning sequence in PBL compared to physicians' activities, 81-84

Mechanics before the group undertakes a problem, 55
Memorization as opposed to understanding, x, 26-29, 84, 97, 127
Memory structures in the physicianís mind, 27
Metacognitive skills, 18
Modified essay question (MEQ), 102
Multiple choice questions (MCQ), 101

Objectives for PBL, 33-36, 78-81

P4 problem simulation, 1
Patient problem characteristics, 7-11
Patients, 44
Pathologies in clinical reasoning, 19-22
Problem boxes, 1, 112
Problem simulations, 12, 40-41
PBL as a simulation of clinical practice, 81-84
PBL in clerkships, x, 1, 111-117
PBL process, 48-88
Problems, choosing, 85, 121-124
Project for learning resource design, 1

Reanalysis of the problem in the light of new information acquired in the PBL process, 68-70, 84

Reasoning of scientists and physicians compared, 19
Reasoning pathologies, 19-22
Resource critique, 67-68
Resource faculty (consultants), 39-40, 66, 67

Schedules, 46-47, 96
Second session with a problem, 67-80
Self and peer assessment, 75-77
Self assessment, 31, 77
Self-directed learning, 50, 62, 65, 66
Self-monitoring, 30
Sequential management problems, 102
Socratic skills as opposed to facilitatory of the tutor, 114
Standardized (simulated) patients, 43, 103-105, 112
Summarizing what has been learned, 59, 70-73

Teacher centered curricula, 35, 85, 95, 107, 114, 122
Teachers concerns about PBL, 85-88
Tests that stress memorization, 87
Transfer of learning to new problems, 73
Tutors, 37, 39, 49-51
Tutor training, 37, 91

Variables that can alter the effectiveness of PBL, 91-97
Varieties of PBL, 2, 34-36